T0291975

Fast Facts for the NEW NURSE PRACTITIONER: *What You Really Need to Know in a Nutshell, 2e* (Aktan)

Fast Facts for the ER NURSE: *Emergency Room Orientation in a Nutshell, 2e* (Buettner)

Fast Facts for the MEDICAL–SURGICAL NURSE: *Clinical Orientation in a Nutshell* (Ciocco)

Fast Facts for the OPERATING ROOM NURSE: *An Orientation and Care Guide in a Nutshell* (Criscitelli)

Fast Facts for the ANTEPARTUM AND POSTPARTUM NURSE: *A Nursing Orientation and Care Guide in a Nutshell* (Davidson)

Fast Facts for the NEONATAL NURSE: *A Nursing Orientation and Care Guide in a Nutshell* (Davidson)

Fast Facts About PRESSURE ULCER CARE FOR NURSES: *How to Prevent, Detect, and Resolve Them in a Nutshell* (Dziedzic)

Fast Facts for the GERONTOLOGY NURSE: *A Nursing Care Guide in a Nutshell* (Eliopoulos)

Fast Facts for the CLINICAL NURSE MANAGER: *Managing a Changing Workplace in a Nutshell* (Fry)

Fast Facts for EVIDENCE-BASED PRACTICE: *Implementing EBP in a Nutshell* (Godshall)

Fast Facts About NURSING AND THE LAW: *Law for Nurses in a Nutshell* (Grant, Ballard)

Fast Facts for the L&D NURSE: *Labor & Delivery Orientation in a Nutshell* (Groll)

Fast Facts for the RADIOLOGY NURSE: *An Orientation and Nursing Care Guide in a Nutshell* (Grossman)

Fast Facts on ADOLESCENT HEALTH FOR NURSING AND HEALTH PROFESSIONALS: *A Care Guide in a Nutshell* (Herrman)

Fast Facts for the FAITH COMMUNITY NURSE: *Implementing FCN/Parish Nursing in a Nutshell* (Hickman)

Fast Facts for the CARDIAC SURGERY NURSE: *Everything You Need to Know in a Nutshell* (Hodge)

Fast Facts for the CLINICAL NURSING INSTRUCTOR: *Clinical Teaching in a Nutshell, 2e* (Kan, Stabler-Haas)

Fast Facts for the WOUND CARE NURSE: *Practical Wound Management in a Nutshell* (Kifer)

Fast Facts About EKGs FOR NURSES: *The Rules of Identifying EKGs in a Nutshell* (Landrum)

Fast Facts for the CRITICAL CARE NURSE: *Critical Care Nursing in a Nutshell* (Landrum)

Fast Facts for the TRAVEL NURSE: *Travel Nursing in a Nutshell* (Landrum)

Fast Facts for the SCHOOL NURSE: *School Nursing in a Nutshell, 2e* (Loschiavo)

Fast Facts About CURRICULUM DEVELOPMENT IN NURSING: *How to Develop & Evaluate Educational Programs in a Nutshell* (McCoy, Anema)

Fast Facts for DEMENTIA CARE: *What Nurses Need to Know in a Nutshell* (Miller)

Fast Facts for HEALTH PROMOTION IN NURSING: *Promoting Wellness in a Nutshell* (Miller)

Fast Facts for STROKE CARE NURSING: *An Expert Guide in a Nutshell* (Morrison)

Fast Facts for the MEDICAL OFFICE NURSE: *What You Really Need to Know in a Nutshell* (Richmeier)

Fast Facts for the PEDIATRIC NURSE: *An Orientation Guide in a Nutshell* (Rupert, Young)

Fast Facts About the GYNECOLOGICAL EXAM FOR NURSE PRACTITIONERS: *Conducting the GYN Exam in a Nutshell* (Secor, Fantasia)

Fast Facts for the STUDENT NURSE: *Nursing Student Success in a Nutshell* (Stabler-Haas)

Fast Facts for CAREER SUCCESS IN NURSING: *Making the Most of Mentoring in a Nutshell* (Vance)

Fast Facts for DEVELOPING A NURSING ACADEMIC PORTFOLIO: *What You Really Need to Know in a Nutshell* (Wittmann-Price)

Fast Facts for the CLASSROOM NURSING INSTRUCTOR: *Classroom Teaching in a Nutshell* (Yoder-Wise, Kowalski)

Forthcoming FAST FACTS Books

Fast Facts for the NURSE PRECEPTOR: *Keys to a Successful Orientation in a Nutshell* (Ciocco)

Fast Facts for the LONG-TERM CARE NURSE: *A Guide for Nurses in Nursing Homes and Assisted Living Settings* (Eliopoulos)

Fast Facts for the CLINICAL NURSE MANAGER: *Managing a Changing Workplace in a Nutshell, 2e* (Fry)

Fast Facts for EVIDENCE-BASED PRACTICE: *Implementing EBP in a Nutshell, 2e* (Godshall)

Fast Facts for the L & D NURSE: *Labor and Delivery Orientation in a Nutshell, 2e* (Groll)

Fast Facts for the CARDIAC SURGERY NURSE: *Caring for Cardiac Surgery Patients in a Nutshell, 2e* (Hodge)

Fast Facts About the NURSING PROFESSION: *Historical Perspectives in a Nutshell* (Hunt)

Fast Facts for the TRIAGE NURSE: *An Orientation and Care Guide in a Nutshell* (Visser, Montejano, Grossman)

Visit www.springerpub.com to order.

FAST FACTS FOR THE
NEW NURSE PRACTITIONER

Nadine M. Aktan, PhD, RN, FNP-BC, received her bachelor's, master's, and doctoral degrees in nursing from Rutgers University College of Nursing and Graduate School in New Brunswick and Newark, New Jersey. She is currently chairperson and associate professor at William Paterson University in Wayne, New Jersey, teaching future nurses and nurse practitioners. She also practices as a family nurse practitioner at the Immedicenter, an urgent care/family practice with locations in Clifton, Bloomfield, and Totowa, New Jersey, and as a maternal–child community health nurse for Valley Home Care in Paramus, New Jersey.

FAST FACTS FOR THE NEW NURSE PRACTITIONER

What You Really Need to Know in a Nutshell

Second Edition

Nadine M. Aktan, PhD, RN, FNP-BC

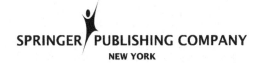

SPRINGER PUBLISHING COMPANY
NEW YORK

Springer Publishing Company, LLC
11 West 42nd Street
New York, NY 10036
www.springerpub.com

Acquisitions Editor: Margaret Zuccarini
Production Editor: Kris Parrish
Composition: S4Carlisle Publishing Services

ISBN: 978-0-8261-3042-6
E-book ISBN: 978-0-8261-3043-3

15 16 17 18 / 5 4 3 2 1

The author and the publisher of this Work have made every effort to use sources believed to be reliable to provide information that is accurate and compatible with the standards generally accepted at the time of publication. The author and publisher shall not be liable for any special, consequential, or exemplary damages resulting, in whole or in part, from the readers' use of, or reliance on, the information contained in this book. The publisher has no responsibility for the persistence or accuracy of URLs for external or third-party Internet websites referred to in this publication and does not guarantee that any content on such websites is, or will remain, accurate or appropriate.

Library of Congress Cataloging-in-Publication Data

Aktan, Nadine M., author.
  Fast facts for the new nurse practitioner : what you really need to know in a nutshell / Nadine M. Aktan.—Second edition.
    p. ; cm.
  Includes bibliographical references and index.
  ISBN 978-0-8261-3042-6—ISBN 978-0-8261-3043-3 (e-book)
  I. Title.
  [DNLM: 1. Nurse Practitioners—United States. 2. Career Choice—United States. 3. Practice Management—United States. 4. Vocational Guidance—United States. WY 128]
  RT82.8
  610.7306'92—dc23
                                                                              2014047654

Printed in the United States of America by Gasch Printing.

Contents

Part X: You're in Charge

Part XI: Economics, Policy, and Future Practice

Foreword

In 1965, Dr. Loretta Ford, a registered nurse (RN), and Dr. Henry Silva, a physician, proposed the nurse practitioner (NP) as another provider model, and its evolution continues. Practices affecting issues of educational preparation, licensure, autonomy, certification, scope of practice, prescriptive authority, and reimbursement still vary among states. Efforts to standardize these practices proceed, so that the maximum benefits of the NP provider to the health care system can be fully realized. When Dr. Nadine Aktan invited me to write the foreword for her book, I wondered how much reference to these ongoing efforts would actually help the reader. As I read each section, however, it became clear that such discussions benefit all readers.

This book teaches you about becoming an NP and invites you to consider topics of importance to both NP students and engaged NPs. Aktan presents information that will help any nursing student or professional RN considering an NP career engage in sound decision making. The reader learns quickly what is really involved in the NP role. There is thoughtful emphasis on the benefits of spending time in examining the "fit" among one's finances, learning style, nonnegotiable life roles, and the demands that accompany preparing for this new career. Also, the reader will acquire some very practical tips on how to maximize learning from the preceptor–student practice experiences that are part of all programs.

Both prospective and established practitioners will benefit from attention to the challenges and rewards that accompany the reality of practice. Because the examples derive from real practice, Atkan's commentary and reflections have a direct, genuine, and practical quality. Her inclusion of possible scenarios portraying intra- and interprofessional dynamics offers a guide to successfully managing these evolving relationships. And her discussion of achieving comfort with the changing responsibilities inherent in this provider role offers valuable insight to NP students, as well as existing practitioners.

The last two sections focus on a selected range of topics and issues of importance to NPs, including questions about why reimbursement schedules for the same patient service can vary by health plan depending on whether the provider is an NP or a physician; commentary on the contribution of NPs to health care and the future impact to be realized from this provider group; and a reasoned discussion of the doctor of nursing practice (DNP) recommendation as the required educational credential for nurse practitioner licensure as of 2015.

This book is well organized, purposeful, and highly readable. It guides the reader through essential material that will contribute to informed decisions. Dr. Aktan's easy and personable style makes the reading enjoyable, and her dual perspective of practicing NP and nurse educator enhances its value. I thank her for the opportunity to share my appreciation of her contribution to those who will benefit from her work.

Kathleen A. Connolly, MEd, RN, APRN-BC
Associate Professor
William Paterson University
Wayne, New Jersey

Preface

My vision for this second edition of this book was to create something I wish had been available when I became a new nurse practitioner (NP). I love being an NP, and I take pride in my discipline. I hope that this contribution to the field will encourage more nurses to consider becoming NPs and that it will also help the next generation of NPs transition more effectively into the role.

The book provides a wealth of information to support you through this journey. It is based on fact and guided by opinion. Yet, overall, its intention is to promote self-reflection, as many of the choices you will make during this process are entirely personal.

This book fills a void for students and newly certified NPs alike, serving as a "guide" or a "manual" in that it incorporates the author's experiences as a family NP and nurse educator. No such other book exists. Until now, all of the information that a student NP or new NP would need was available only in many different places—not in one reputable and convenient source. This is the resource that any nurse considering becoming an NP needs, and any student or new NP must have. The second edition includes five new chapters and many updates throughout.

Recent literature on the history of the NP role is explored and explained, but this is not a traditional textbook. Humor and real-life clinical examples are included. Useful tips and resources, such as professional organizations, networks, associations, and websites, are shared with the reader. Most importantly, the reader is provided with insight from experts in the field in a "What You Really Need to Know" format.

The role of the NP is a hot topic in today's ever-changing, ever-challenging, and economically driven health care system. Newer nurses, in increasing numbers, are being encouraged to enroll in nursing graduate programs sooner than they ever were before to fulfill this increasing need. This trend will continue to accelerate because of current and future health care demands and the economic benefits NPs offer.

Although NPs have been around for decades, only recently has our role become an essential component in meeting society's health care demands. This book explores reasons to become an NP, provides insight on issues related to NP education, clarifies hot topics related to NP practice, and proposes how the role of the NP is continuing to evolve. This is the all-in-one reference for potential or current NP students as well as newly practicing NPs. Its chapters contain learning objectives, checklists to facilitate important decision making, charts and tables highlighting hot topics or key elements, and testimonials from currently practicing NPs, as well as the author's own poignant moments as a new and experienced NP that will be helpful to any new or soon-to-be-new practitioner. Significant points are set in boldface type throughout, and pertinent information is summarized in boxes that offer "Fast Facts in a Nutshell."

Nadine M. Aktan

Acknowledgments

I sat down to write this book for two reasons—to create something I wish had been available to me as a new NP and to give back to a profession that has given so much to me. As health care professionals, we have the ability to heal. We have the ability to help. We have the ability to empower others and make a difference each and every day. This book is for my present and future NP colleagues. I hope that this resource will help you through the bureaucracy of the health care system, so that you can focus all of your efforts on your patients. After all, is that not what it is all about?

I want to acknowledge my many teachers, preceptors, mentors, colleagues, students, and friends in the discipline of nursing. Thank you to my precious Delila and Jett for inspiring me to strive to do better each and every day; to my husband, Mukbil, for your love and support and for being my best friend; to my mother, Barbara, for shaping me into the woman I am today; and to my incredible, supportive family and wonderful friends for all you do for me.

PART

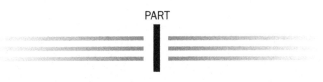

I

Making the Decision

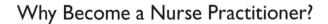

Why Become a Nurse Practitioner?

You are a registered nurse (RN), who is considering attending graduate school to become a nurse practitioner (NP). Maybe you have worked closely with one of these nurse experts. Possibly, you are just ready for a change— or even a challenge!

This chapter discusses the role of the NP, why you might want to pursue such a career, and what steps are necessary to achieve this goal. It explains the different degrees available, such as the master's-prepared NP and the doctor of nursing practice (DNP). Finally, it explores the current and future role of the NP, the job market, and the many benefits the job offers.

In this chapter, you will learn:

1. An overview of the role of the NP
2. The reasons to become an NP
3. Recommendations on how to pursue this career path

THE ROLE OF THE NURSE PRACTITIONER

The current role of the NP is to provide expert nursing care. In addition, an NP often adopts a medical approach to patient care, as **NPs have the authority to assess, diagnose, and treat patients in a variety of settings.**

What are NPs allowed to do? This varies from state to state. In general, most NPs function as the primary health care providers for their clients. **NPs can order tests, prescribe medications, and refer patients to specialty providers.** They manage their own patients and follow up as necessary. If patients require care above and beyond an NP's scope of practice, the NP refers them to a physician colleague. For additional information about the role of the NP, see Chapter 13.

FAST FACTS in a NUTSHELL

- NPs provide expert nursing care.
- NPs function as the primary health care providers for their patients.

REASONS TO BECOME A NURSE PRACTITIONER

I chose to become an NP for many reasons—personal and professional growth, a greater sense of autonomy, higher salary potential, and increased job satisfaction. In addition, there was my response to a question that made my skin crawl: "You are so smart, why didn't you just become a doctor?" I am sure many, if not most, of you reading this book have been asked this question. My response is simple: "Because I love being a nurse." Nurses have the unusual ability to combine medical knowledge with a holistic approach to patient care.

Although many NPs function in a role that is, at times, similar to that of physicians, we do so differently because we look at our patients differently. Nursing is our art, and NPs take nursing care to the next level.

Why are you becoming an NP? Whether your reasons are the same as mine or are your own, deciding to make the change is the first step. You must then discover the steps necessary to achieve this goal.

Some reasons to become an NP are professional growth, autonomy, an increase in salary, and greater job satisfaction.

THE FIRST STEP

The first step in deciding to pursue a graduate degree is to do your research. Ask NPs what they like and dislike about the NP role. Consider your interests—both now and in the future.

Review the job market in your area. From job posting sites, you will likely discover positions available in a practice or institution near you. Familiarize yourself with the potential salary ranges that have been reported, from $64,100 to $120,500 annually (U.S. News & World Report, "Nurse Practitioner: Salary," n.d.), and the other benefits the position will offer (see Chapter 18). Although the job market varies from region to region, there is an overall strong national demand for NPs.

Explore the differences between master's-prepared NPs and those who have earned a doctor of nursing practice (DNP) degree. Understand how NPs differ from other types of advanced practice nurses (APNs)—the clinical nurse specialist, certified nurse midwife, and certified registered nurse anesthetist. The DNP, the most advanced degree for nursing practice, will be described in greater detail in Chapter 30.

≡ *FAST FACTS in a NUTSHELL*

The first steps in considering becoming an NP:

- Talk to some NPs.
- Review the job market in your area.
- Learn the differences between the master's-prepared NP and the doctor of nursing practice (DNP).

Many of you may ask about the differences between an NP and a physician's assistant (PA). The answer is simple: prior experience and education. **An NP has previous nursing experience as an RN.** Therefore, NPs share basic nursing knowledge and skills; they are experts in the art of caring and the science of medicine. On the other hand, a PA may or may not have previous health care experience or education in health care science.

Still, in many practice sites, the roles performed by the NP and the PA can seem similar—even, at times, identical, depending on what needs to be done. The actual scope of practice for the NP and the PA, however, differs state by state.

=== *FAST FACTS in a NUTSHELL*

As you consider a career as an NP, keep in mind this excerpt written by a former nursing student who is now studying to become an NP: *At one point in my nursing school career I considered leaving the field of nursing and heading to medical school because I was not sure of the scope and the ability of the NP. After working with NPs in the field, I realized that I could do everything I wanted to as a family nurse practitioner (FNP). I do not want it to sound like I settled for becoming an NP—far from it. I just realized that the FNP role would fit me better than the MD role.*

2

How to Begin

Various nurse practitioner (NP) specialty areas are available for certification. Selecting the correct one for you may be easy or may pose some challenges. This chapter guides you through the first step in this journey. First, it is essential that you understand the types of NP specialties available. Then, you should follow some recommended guidelines in deciding which is right for you. Good ways to begin include incorporating your nursing background and experiences, spending time with experts in the field, and reflecting on future career goals.

In this chapter, you will learn:

1. The types of NP specialties offered
2. How to decide which is best for you

NURSING PRACTITIONER SPECIALTIES

New or potential NPs may consider a variety of areas for certification, including acute care, adult–gerontology, family, pediatric, psychiatric, women's health, neonatal, and occupational health. Here, your educational background and nursing experience can play an important role in selecting your specialty. For instance, what population(s) have you worked with as a nurse? Which did you most (or least) enjoy? Have there been any area(s) of nursing that you always dreamed of working in? Newer nurses may also consider their student clinical rotations to help answer some of these questions.

My own experience provides an example of how you can begin to select an NP specialty. My hospital-based nursing experience was primarily in pediatrics in a large, urban medical center. Early on, I knew hospital nursing was not quite right for me. After gaining acute care experience, I found a better fit. I moved out of the hospital into the field of maternal–child community health nursing. Here, I also did some work in pediatric hospice, where I participated in the development and implementation of a pediatric hospice program.

When I decided to pursue my master's degree, I initially considered becoming a pediatric nurse practitioner (PNP). However, community health nursing had been such a powerful experience for me. I also had great interest in women's health. I was faced with the decision of choosing a specific population to work with or selecting a broader area of certification.

I was not certain that I wanted to commit to just one NP specialty. This is why family practice was an appealing option for me. For an additional six credits and 100 or so clinical hours, I could legally practice in providing care for individuals in all age groups. I felt this would be the best fit, as it would incorporate my areas of interest at that time, while leaving the door open for others in the future.

FAST FACTS in a NUTSHELL

Some areas for certification include acute care, adult–gerontology, family, pediatric, psychiatric, women's health, neonatal, and occupational health.

WHAT IS RIGHT FOR YOU?

I made the right choice for myself. Over more than 15 years of experience in family practice, I have managed the acute and chronic health care needs of patients ranging from newborns to those older than 100 years. I learn something new every day that I practice. That is what makes my clinical work exciting for me. Every day is different. Every day is a challenge. Every day is an adventure!

However, I do not recommend this approach for everyone. Some of you have a special ability to work with newborns, for example, or the elderly. This is your passion. I do not recommend choosing a broader specialty when you know deep inside exactly where your calling is. I believe that the decision to pursue a new avenue in your nursing career is so personal that you really need to reflect on your experiences as well as your career goals as you choose.

I recommend spending time with practitioners in the specialty areas you are considering. I take nursing students with me into my NP practice for observational experiences all the time. I have never had one end the day without a newly discovered passion to go on to graduate school.

═══════════════*FAST FACTS in a NUTSHELL*

In deciding on an NP specialty area, you need to reflect on your past nursing experiences, as well as your future career goals.

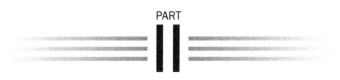

PART

II

Selecting an Educational Program

3

Types of Programs

One of the most important decisions you will make in your graduate nursing career is selecting a nurse practitioner (NP) program. It is through your graduate education that you will develop the essential skills and knowledge base for NP practice. Yet, possibly even more important, it is here that you will create your personal NP philosophy.

This chapter guides your exploration of the various types of NP programs available. You are encouraged to consider a number of factors relevant to determining the quality of and selecting an NP program.

In this chapter, you will learn:

1. The types of NP programs available
2. How to select an NP program
3. Ways to evaluate an NP program

WHICH TYPE OF PROGRAM IS RIGHT FOR YOU?

Once you decide to become an NP, **the next step is to carefully** explore the various types of programs available.

Today, an NP student has the luxury of choosing from more than 800 programs in more than 350 schools. He or she can consider local or hybrid (a blend of online and face-to-face courses) programs. For some online programs, students do not have to be within close geographical proximity of the institution. Students in all programs use technology to interact with faculty and peers; face-to-face interaction takes place in the clinical setting.

Before you decide, think about what type of learner you are. Do you need face-to-face interaction? Are you tech savvy, or are you willing to become so? What about other commitments, such as work schedule, economics, and personal or family obligations? Many of these factors may not have been as influential when you were an undergraduate student as they are now.

I am an avid supporter of online education. I teach online courses to undergraduate and graduate students, and have taken online courses myself. If properly developed and implemented, including thoughtful consideration to how students can effectively meet course objectives, online courses are a valid means of preparing students in a variety of career paths.

Yet, with this being said, I value face-to-face interactions. Student interaction with faculty and peers in a traditional classroom setting is a meaningful part of the educational experience. Therefore, I encourage a blend of classroom, online, and clinical courses to best prepare you for your future NP practice. Many reputable online programs successfully prepare NP graduates. As with anything, the right program coupled with the right student will result in success.

Consider the following criteria to help you in deciding on a type of nursing graduate program that meets your individualized needs (traditional, hybrid, online):

I enjoy technology.	Yes/No
I am open to new ways of learning.	Yes/No
I have a busy schedule (work, personal commitments).	Yes/No

I am focused and budget my time well.   Yes/No

I work well independently and in groups.   Yes/No

I am in interested in a program that is a great
    geographical distance from where I live, and   Yes/No

I am not interested in relocating.   Yes/No

If you answered yes to three or more of these statements, hybrid or online education might be something for you to consider.

════════════════════════*FAST FACTS in a NUTSHELL*

- In determining what type of program is right for you, consider what type of learner you are.
- A blend of classroom, online, and clinical courses may best prepare you for your future NP practice.

STEPS FOR SUCCESS

All of these factors and many more come into play as you embark on this journey. After narrowing down potential programs—at both the master's and doctoral levels—make appointments with directors of the various programs you are considering. Inquire about opportunities to meet faculty, current students, and alumnae. Explore their individual curricula, academic policies, and potential clinical placements. In addition, find out about the library, resources, and other forms of student support services available.

Then gather information on the quality of each program. You do so primarily by examining program credentials and success rates on certification examinations (more on this below). Another prudent step is to research potential employers' opinions of the programs you are considering. Much of this information may come from those nursing colleagues and mentors you will be encouraged to identify in Chapter 7. Some of it may come from other professionals, such as physicians, administrators, and recruiters.

========================= *FAST FACTS in a NUTSHELL*

- Explore various programs directly and by talking to experts in the field.
- Gather information on the quality of each program.

EVALUATING A PROGRAM

There are several other things I encourage you to look for when considering a program. Most importantly, a potential student must consider whether a program is accredited. Accreditation is extremely important. This truly speaks to the quality of the program. It may also be a factor in whether or not a program's graduates are eligible to take the various certification exams.

In addition, find out how long has the program been in existence. What are the program's certification pass rates? I would be leery of a program that is unable or unwilling to share these data. You want to know that if you successfully complete a program, you will pass your boards!

========================= *FAST FACTS in a NUTSHELL*

- Consider whether a program is accredited.
- Find out how long a program has been in existence.
- What are the program's certification pass rates?

Something for a potential student to consider is program rankings. *U.S. News & World Report* (2011) rated the top nursing graduate programs on the basis of the results of peer assessment surveys sent to deans, other administrators, and faculty at accredited degree programs. Schools with the top rankings in some of the specialty practice areas are listed in Table 3.1. Additional information can be found online (http://grad-schools.usnews.rankingsandreviews.com/best-graduate-schools/top-health-schools/nursing-rankings?int=992108).

TABLE 3.1 Top NP Program Rankings

Adult
University of Pennsylvania
University of California, San Francisco and University of Washington
Columbia University and University of Michigan, Ann Arbor
University of Pittsburgh
Rush University
University of Maryland, Baltimore
Yale University
Duke University and University of Alabama, Birmingham

Family
University of California, San Francisco
University of Washington
University of Pennsylvania
University of Michigan, Ann Arbor
Columbia University
Oregon Health and Science University
Johns Hopkins University
Yale University
University of Maryland, Baltimore
Vanderbilt University

Pediatric
University of Pennsylvania
Yale University
University of Washington
University of Pittsburgh
Duke University
Rush University
University of Colorado, Denver
University of California, San Francisco
Columbia University
University of North Carolina, Chapel Hill

Data from *U.S. News & World Report* (2011).

SELECTING THE RIGHT PROGRAM FOR YOU

Although Table 3.1 includes a rather prestigious list of top-notch academic institutions, I do not want you to think that these are the only good programs available. You certainly do not have to attend one of these programs to have a thriving NP career.

As an example, I will describe the program in which I currently teach. It is a relatively small, solid, and reputable program located at a university in northwest New Jersey not far from New York City. An adult–gerontology NP program and a family NP program are offered. The doctor of nursing practice (DNP) program is the first doctoral program at our university.

The program is fully accredited and boasts a history of consistently high certification pass rates. The faculty is committed and diverse; its members work closely with the student population from the first theory course right through to the completion of the final thesis project. The faculty has vast clinical contacts, and student feedback on the program is extremely positive.

I recently sat in a room full of graduate students and asked them what they liked or disliked about the program. Overwhelmingly, the consensus was that they appreciated how well they got to know their classmates and their faculty throughout their graduate years. According to the members of this group, they found the faculty to be approachable and engaging—always knowing their names and easy to get in touch with.

Is this important to you? If not, what is? Remember the process of self-reflection I referred to earlier? This is one time when this step is critical.

═══════════════════════════*FAST FACTS in a NUTSHELL*

The take-home message is this: Some students do well in large programs, others in smaller ones. Some require high levels of faculty and student engagement; others do not. Think about the positive and not-so-positive attributes of your undergraduate nursing experience. These may be helpful in fostering the decision-making process.

4

Scholarships, Resources, and More

Let's face it: Tuition is not cheap. When you consider the different salaries of nurses and nurse practitioners (NPs), part of the decision-making equation must account for the cost of graduate education. A wealth of information is available to those who search for it. If your employer will not fully fund your tuition, you should make every effort to research scholarships, grants, and other programs.

This chapter discusses the potential costs of graduate education—beyond tuition alone. It also guides you through some possible means of funding graduate studies. Potential resources and helpful suggestions for funding are provided. The overall recommendation to the reader is to be creative, be innovative, and to think "outside the box."

In this chapter, you will learn:

1. The costs of a graduate education
2. Ways to fund, in part or in full, graduate studies
3. Ideas, websites, and other resources that can provide practical information

HOW MUCH WILL IT ALL COST?

The answer to this question varies. Just as with your undergraduate education, tuition and associated fees vary from state to state and from institution to institution. Before you apply for any program, find out exactly what the cost will be. It would be quite unfortunate not to complete a program in which you are enrolled because of unanticipated costs.

Costs include more than tuition. Be prepared to pay for textbooks, fees for clinical courses, access to computer programs and simulation models, a higher level of malpractice insurance, lab coats, and possibly other pieces of equipment, such as otoscopes and ophthalmoscopes.

Be aware of the possibility of lost wages. Once an NP student begins clinical courses, he or she will be responsible for completing a certain number of clinical hours per week or per semester (to be discussed more in Chapter 6). This may mean that the student must work fewer hours and, therefore, receive less pay. In return, through the clinical practical experience, the student will receive support toward the attainment of clinical skills and knowledge, role development, competence, and confidence.

Many students seem surprised when they realize the expectations for clinical hours and related coursework. Graduate school is a commitment. It costs time and it costs money. This needs to be factored in to your decision-making process. Your success in an NP program and overall in the field is dependent upon your understanding these important factors right from the start.

═══════════FAST FACTS in a NUTSHELL

The cost of NP education includes tuition, fees, books and other materials, clinical fees, malpractice insurance, uniforms, equipment, and lost wages.

Before you go any further, become an expert in your employer's tuition reimbursement programs and opportunities. In most cases, larger hospitals and institutions will support their nurses in full or in part to enable them to continue their nursing education. If yours does not, ask! You may be able to negotiate for full or partial tuition reimbursement in some smaller institutions or practices.

If your employer will not completely fund your education, then it is up to you to explore opportunities for funding. Grants, scholarships, traineeships, and a variety of other programs may be just what you are looking for. Most likely, the Internet is the best place to begin. Table 4.1 provides a list of useful websites.

Of course, this list is not all-inclusive—not even close! Meet with career counselors. Search the web. Think "outside the box." For example, consider future work with indigent populations or persons from other underdeveloped or underserved areas. Some programs will offer to pay part of your tuition if you agree to work in areas lacking adequate numbers of health care providers.

TABLE 4.1 Useful Resources

Advanced Education Nursing Traineeship (www.bhpr.hrsa.gov/nursing/grants/aent.html)

American Association of Colleges of Nursing (www.aacn.nche.edu/students/financial-aid)

American Association of Nurse Practitioners (www.aanp.org/practice/grants-scholarships2)

American Nurse Practitioner Foundation (www.anp-foundation.org/programs/scholarships-grants/funding/)

Federal Nurse Traineeship (www.federalgrantswire.com/advanced-education-nursing-traineeships.html)

Minority Nurse (www.minoritynurse.com/find-scholarships)

National Health Service Corps (www.nhsc.hrsa.gov/scholarships/)

===== *FAST FACTS in a NUTSHELL*

- Grants, scholarships, traineeships, and a variety of other programs are available to those who apply for them.
- Consider future work in underserved areas to pay for part of your tuition.

WHAT TO APPLY FOR

This point cannot be overemphasized: *Apply for everything for which you are eligible.* Even though I was a practicing nurse in an institution that provided some tuition reimbursement, I found that attending graduate school full time made me eligible for a federal program that covered three out of four semesters of graduate school. It even provided a stipend for textbooks. **Do not assume that you may not qualify to receive full or partial financial support for your education.** I was lucky enough to have the majority of my education funded by employers, traineeships, and grants because I took the time to look and apply.

===== *FAST FACTS in a NUTSHELL*

- Students should apply for everything for which they are eligible.
- Do not assume that you will not qualify for financial support.

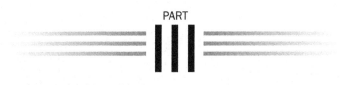

PART

III

Finding the Right Clinical Preceptor

5

Important Things to Consider

Choosing the right clinical preceptors are some of the most important decisions you will make during graduate study. It is the time spent in clinical training that will truly teach you how to perform as a practicing nurse practitioner (NP). Selecting an effective preceptor is the first step to success on your journey. This decision has a direct effect on your early years in practice.

This chapter discusses factors you should consider in selecting the right clinical preceptor for you. Practical ways to maximize clinical opportunities are also emphasized. Once you have selected a preceptor, it is time to prepare and to begin!

In this chapter, you will learn:

1. Factors related to selecting the best clinical preceptors
2. Pitfalls to avoid
3. How to adequately prepare for the clinical experience

HOW, WHAT, AND WHERE

Some graduate programs will arrange for a student's clinical experience. Most will guide the NP student in the process of identifying and securing the best placements, with the student taking the lead in this process. Often, students will receive a list of potential acceptable preceptors who have been used by their institution's department in the past and who meet guidelines set by accrediting bodies.

The best approach for the student is to select a preceptor from a list of previously approved practitioners. This way the student can work in and gain experience from areas in which he or she is interested—and, possibly, even find mentors or land a future job!

Only you know what your ultimate career goals are. A student who selects a preceptor in his or her own personal area of interest benefits most from the experience. This generally works out better than when a particular preceptor is assigned to an NP student. Students may not recognize or understand this initially but likely will in the end.

Of course, geographical location and the preceptor's hours of availability are important elements in this consideration. However, you should also consider other factors. The expertise one gains during the required 500- or 600-plus clinical hours is paramount in the effective transition to the role of NP. Do not waste this valuable time simply because of convenience in scheduling.

A good place to start is by seeking advice from faculty, peers, colleagues, and other mentors in the field. Who were their preceptors? Who was the best? Who was not that great? Their feedback will start you in the right direction. Be sure to inquire about a variety of potential preceptor types—for example, NPs and physicians. Spend time with these different types of expert clinicians to make the most of these supervised hours.

═══════════════════════════*FAST FACTS in a NUTSHELL*

- To find a good fit, students should select their own preceptors from a list of previously approved practitioners who meet the guidelines set by accrediting bodies.
- A good place to start is by seeking advice from faculty peers, colleagues, and other mentors in the field.

Consider varying your experiences and populations based on your interests—actual or potential. Then participate in completing the required hours in a variety of settings, both inpatient and outpatient. Some examples of locations and settings in which to identify and secure a variety of quality preceptors include, but are not limited to, hospitals, private physician offices, urgent care centers, birthing centers, surgical centers, long-term care facilities, managed care organizations, retail clinics, occupational health sites, schools, college health centers, correctional facilities, clinics, and other forms of community outreach.

Spend time in urban, suburban, or rural environments when practical. This exposure is essential to learning about how the NP role varies from setting to setting and from one environment to the next. You will note major differences in the role as you rotate through a multitude of settings.

In addition, consider whether the patients managed by potential preceptors are the types of patients you see yourself working with. For example, if you are enrolled in a women's health NP program but the preceptor you are considering sees both male and female clients, you will not gain the ideal number of patient contacts per clinical hour. Carefully consider the best use of every hour of your clinical time.

While in graduate school, my own clinical experiences varied. During my pediatric rotation, for example, I selected two different preceptors. For the first half of the semester, I worked with a pediatric nurse practitioner (PNP) in a fast-paced inner city practice. During the second half of the semester, my preceptor was a PNP in a suburban private physician practice. What a world of difference!

This semester was an eye-opening experience for me. It was amazing to see how similar diagnoses can be managed differently depending on the patient and family, their insurance or lack of insurance, and a multitude of other factors, such as socioeconomic background and the reliability of family members. I was fortunate to have been able to arrange for this opportunity. Whenever possible, I highly recommend that students make an effort to arrange for similar activities and experiences.

========================*FAST FACTS in a NUTSHELL*

- It is important to vary your clinical experiences and populations based on your interests.
- Participate in completing the required hours in a variety of settings, both inpatient and outpatient.
- Spend time in urban, suburban, or rural environments when practical.

WHAT TO LOOK OUT FOR

I also spent one full semester working with a physician. This was beneficial in many ways. Choosing a physician preceptor may prove useful for you as well. This is not, however, a necessary component of NP education. For me, it was an opportunity to relate NP practice to that of a physician colleague. The drawback for me was that the physician did not fully understand the NP role or my role as a student. I can reflect on this now, but at the time I do not think I handled the situation properly.

Overall, the physician viewed my time there as observational. This is *not* the way to spend your valuable clinical time. Although observation is an acceptable, and even necessary, way to learn your preceptor's style and gain a basic overview of the practice, you should not spend more time than necessary in this role. Mere observation will not prepare you to assume the role of an autonomous practitioner. You need to be an active participant in your learning process. Studies show that a student learns more effectively this way. The NP role is one you will learn by doing and doing and doing. I cannot urge this critical facet of your graduate experience strongly enough.

Although important, observation should be a limited part of the NP student's clinical experience.

GETTING STARTED

So, you have reviewed your options and selected your first preceptor. Now you are ready to get started. Review your objectives—both personal and those set forth in course guidelines provided by faculty. Clarify them with your faculty supervisor when necessary.

Meet with your preceptor in advance when permissible to be sure you will be comfortable working with him or her and also to have the opportunity to see the person in action. This will give you a basic overview of how his or her day works. You will then be able to adequately plan for your experience.

Inquire about the most common types of patients and diagnoses you will encounter. Then prepare. Familiarizing yourself in advance will help you get the most out of every clinical hour. It is during your clinical experience that you have a mentor to fall back on. Once you are out in the real world, you likely will not always have this luxury. The importance of mentorship will be presented in the next chapter.

TEST YOURSELF

Read the following scenario and answer the question that follows to find out what you have learned in this chapter.

Bob is a bright and motivated NP student. He has completed his core courses in an adult–gerontology (AGNP) program and is ready to begin his first clinical course. He consults Susan, his former nursing colleague from the intensive care unit, who is now an experienced NP in an internal medicine practice. Susan recommends four potential preceptors. Which of the following would be the best choice for Bob to pursue as a potential preceptor?

1. Susan herself! They had so much fun working nights together at the hospital. Susan would love to "show him the ropes."
2. Dr. Jones, a physician with whom they both worked in the hospital, who is always looking for an extra set of hands in his busy private practice.
3. Bill, one of Susan's former preceptors, an adult NP who works at a free medical clinic for the indigent. He has been an NP for more than 20 years and is also an adjunct faculty member at another NP program.
4. Kathy, an NP at a retail clinic. She is a new graduate from the same school that Bob attends. This would be an asset because she is familiar with Bob's program.

Correct answer: 3.
In evaluating the possible options, consider the following:

1. Although this choice may be tempting, it is usually not the best idea to select a friend as a preceptor. I cannot stress enough the value of your clinical time. A student may feel comfortable with a preceptor with whom he or she has an existing relationship. Yet, the clinical experience could be adversely affected if the student does not feel sufficiently challenged.
2. An NP student should not be seen as an extra set of hands. A student needs a teacher. Acting as a preceptor to a student takes time! A preceptor who is too busy may not be the best choice.
3. This preceptor seems ideal—highly experienced and a faculty member. Preceptors who are also teachers generally have a better understanding of the objectives to be met by the student.
4. New graduates are still developing their own practices and may not be ready to support a student's development. As a general guideline, an NP should be ready to be a preceptor after at least 1 year of practice. In addition, retail

clinics see many pediatric clients. Therefore, this may not be an appropriate clinical site for an AGNP student.

━━━━━━━━━━━━━━━*FAST FACTS in a NUTSHELL*

Ask your preceptor about the most common patients and diagnoses you will encounter so that you can adequately prepare for your clinical experience.

6

Balancing It All

You have started! You have selected a top program, been accepted, and have enrolled. You rearranged your schedule and have begun taking your core classes. You are doing well and have maintained an acceptable grade point average (GPA). You cannot believe how much you have learned in such a short time and that you actually might be ready to begin to apply this body of knowledge in your first clinical rotation. One question remains: How will you balance it all?

This chapter presents the overall expectations for clinical courses. Some concepts related to balancing work and other commitments and completing the required clinical hours are discussed. Basic ideas for immersion in the NP "culture," as well as a variety of ways to get started, are presented.

In this chapter, you will learn:

1. Basic guidelines for clinical expectations
2. How to successfully manage clinical time
3. Tips for clinical immersion and seeking guidance

WHAT WILL YOU DO DURING THE CLINICAL EXPERIENCE?

Think back to nursing school. During the first year or two, you learned a great deal about nursing and medicine. You listened to experienced faculty. You likely watched a variety of videos and participated in simulation activities. Yet frankly, where did you learn how to perform nursing activities? It was by participating in baccalaureate-level clinical courses. The process during your NP training will be somewhat similar, yet also different.

Clinical training is where you actually learn the NP role. You have been guided through the major concepts of the role in your theory and related core courses. However, it is by working alongside your preceptor that you actually begin to assume the role of the novice NP.

The required number of clinical hours ranges from 500 to 600 throughout graduate study, depending on the type of NP certification. A family nurse practitioner (FNP), for example, is required to complete at least 600 hours because of the nature of the experiences required, whereas the adult–gerontology nurse practitioner (AGNP) student is mandated to complete a minimum of 500 hours. This requirement is divided among the semesters of clinical courses (likely between 120 and 190 clinical hours per semester).

As you can see, this mandate translates into approximately 10 to 12 clinical hours per week. As always, the specifics may vary from program to program. Gather information on requirements for clinical hours before considering an NP program.

═══════════════════════════════ *FAST FACTS in a NUTSHELL*

- It is by working alongside your preceptor that you actually begin to assume the role of the novice NP.
- Gather information on clinical hour requirements before considering an NP program.

You may begin to struggle with the number of clinical hours that need to be completed for each course or semester—or even for each week! You are also likely to be concerned with how to narrow the various clinical preceptor possibilities and fit it all into your already busy schedule. I often hear NP students express concerns about successfully juggling work commitments, family and other personal obligations, and clinical hours, along with related coursework.

Balancing it all is not easy. Talk to other NP students or practicing NPs. How did they manage? What are their recommendations for success? We are all living proof that it can be done—although it does take patience, and commitment. Nothing that is truly worthwhile in life is easy, right?

Begin by setting aside consistent blocks of time to spend with your preceptor. Usually, 1 or 2 days a week will facilitate this. Some students choose to complete some of their hours by using vacation time from their jobs. I think this is a great idea and can work out well if done right.

FAST FACTS in a NUTSHELL

Set aside consistent blocks of time to spend with your preceptor.

IMMERSION

Overall, this process is all about immersion. You need to immerse yourself in a new "culture," so to speak. Experts believe that the more time you spend in a particular culture the easier it will be to learn its language, norms, and customs. Therefore, the more time you are able to spend in the clinical setting, with your clinical preceptor to guide you, the more you will become a part of the NP culture. If you interact consistently as "one of the staff" during that semester, they will begin to treat you this way. This may even be helpful when you are looking for a job.

Come up with a plan that you believe will work for you right from the start. Have it approved by your preceptor and your faculty supervisor. For example, if you plan to use some vacation time to immerse yourself in your clinical culture, be certain that your preceptor can commit to working with you during that period. Taking on a student is time and energy consuming. Some preceptors may decide they can only commit to working with a student 1 or 2 days per week.

FAST FACTS in a NUTSHELL

Immerse yourself in the NP culture.

WHO WILL GUIDE YOU?

You have planned your semester and are ready to begin. Where do you start? Your faculty supervisor will provide you with course objectives, but you will probably be required to formulate your own objectives as well. Your preceptor will then guide you through your first steps toward success. Be patient. Be realistic. Work hard.

One practical suggestion for getting started was very useful to me. Create a "cheat sheet." After each clinical day, write out (or key) the most common diagnoses seen, and details of the treatment plan. Do so by making lists or charts or whatever makes most sense to you.

Add the following important information: What medications were prescribed? What tests were ordered? Was the patient referred to a specialist? If so, what type and when? Based on the results, what was the next course of action? You might even begin to keep track of the names of the best specialists used for referrals, as well as some possible locations for imaging centers and other types of diagnostic testing. This can be a tremendous resource for you early in practice. Add to it weekly—then again at the end of each semester.

How does your cheat sheet vary from preceptor to preceptor? Revise it as you go along to make it more comprehensive or user friendly. This will be a useful reference when you begin to practice independently. I kept mine in my pocket for my first few months at my first job—I am not sure how I would have survived without it!

==========*FAST FACTS in a NUTSHELL*

- Be patient. Be realistic. Work hard.
- After each clinical day, write out (or key) the most common diagnoses seen, including details of the treatment plan.

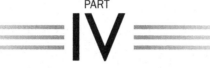

PART

IV

Searching for a Mentor

7

What to Look For

Seeking out quality mentors in the field is important—right from the start! Even though the nurse practitioner (NP) role was established in 1965, the concept is still surprisingly new to some nurses, to other members of the health care community and, even more, to the public. After reading this chapter, you will understand that finding a quality mentor is an essential part of becoming an effective NP.

This chapter discusses the importance of and steps for seeking out mentors. Some personal experiences are shared, and ideas for identifying your own mentors are provided.

In this chapter, you will learn:

1. Why you need a mentor
2. Qualities to look for in a mentor
3. How to establish mentoring relationships

WHAT A MENTOR WILL DO FOR YOU

A good mentor will show you the ropes. Along with your clinical preceptors (some of whom will likely become your future mentors), mentors will guide you through the baby steps of becoming an effective NP in your area of interest. They will introduce you to the people you need to know and what you need to know to get started. I continue to value my mentors and strive to do the best I can to mentor those who will be the future of our profession.

One of my first clinical preceptors became an important mentor for me. Right out of graduate school, I was hired into the same practice where I had obtained my clinical hours as an NP student. I was fortunate to be working alongside my former preceptor, a highly experienced NP to whom I felt comfortable turning when presented with complex clinical questions, during those first months of practice. This situation was ideal for me but may not be practical, or even possible, for all. There are many other ways to find mentors.

Remember your first few months as a nurse? Well many, if not all, of these feelings will come right back when you assume this new role. Not everyone will be quite so lucky as to have a mentor in the same practice. But that is okay. You can talk on the phone, e-mail, or meet for lunch on occasion. Just bouncing ideas off someone who has been through a similar experience will help you through the transition into your new role. Having a mentor you are comfortable with and able to contact when necessary is an invaluable resource.

=== *FAST FACTS in a NUTSHELL*

- Strong mentors will guide you on your journey to becoming an effective NP.
- Mentors will guide you through the baby steps of becoming an effective NP in your area of interest.

QUALITY, BUT ALSO QUANTITY

What qualities should you look for in a mentor? Probably some of the same qualities you looked for in a preceptor, and possibly those you will look for in a collaborating physician.

You need to honestly evaluate your strengths and determine in what areas you will need guidance.

For example, if you have difficulty with delegation, you may call a former preceptor who excelled in this role. If you struggle with ECG interpretation, an NP specializing in cardiology whom you met at a recent conference may become a mentor for you.

Remember, it is great to have mentors right at your side during your first few months of practice. However, this may not be possible. A mentor can be a phone call, text, or e-mail away.

Where should you look? On the job is a good place to start. Even if a mentor is not directly present in your practice setting, he or she may be on staff in other areas of the institution. Other ways to network are through professional organizations and attendance at conferences. Staying in touch with faculty and former classmates is another important way to develop mentors and to mentor one another.

Consider starting an NP group at your institution or with NPs practicing in your area. This is an excellent way to network and support one another in the role. Meet for coffee or lunch once a month.

I even recommend having more than one mentor. Search for someone who is certified in the same area of certification you intend to obtain. Search for mentors who work with the same population (the indigent, for example) or in the same environment (hospital, clinic, or private practice). Search for mentors who are novice NPs. They will likely be aware of exactly how you feel and understand how important their own mentors were (or still are) for them. Search for mentors who are experienced NPs. They will have the most insight from years in practice.

=== *FAST FACTS in a NUTSHELL*

- Consider starting an NP group at your institution or with NPs practicing in your area.
- You can have more than one mentor

THE BENEFITS

What else can I learn from my mentor, you may ask? I often ask my students to consider the difference between "real world" and "textbook" nursing. As students, we learn the textbook way. In practice, sometimes, things are slightly different.

I can remember one of my early mentors in nursing, the charge nurse on the evening shift where I worked in my first position as a pediatric nurse. On a particular day, early on in my orientation, after injecting a frightened and somewhat agitated pediatric patient, she had to quickly move to another important nursing task. To keep herself and the client safe, she stuck the needle into the mattress.

I never heard about this in nursing school! Was she crazy? No. She did what she had to do to prioritize, stabilize the patient, and of course, to protect herself from a needle stick injury. Once she had done so, she safely placed the used needle and syringe into the proper sharps container.

I am certainly not advocating for this practice (safety guidelines from the Occupational Safety and Health Administration [OSHA] and others have since been implemented), but I use this extreme example to demonstrate how what we learn in school is not always exactly what is commonly done in nursing practice. It is no different when you become an NP. Your mentors, preceptors, other NPs, and physicians will play an important role in preparing you for real world practice.

FAST FACTS in a NUTSHELL

A good mentor will teach you what you need to know in preparation for autonomous practice.

8

You as a Mentor

Many of you are likely already mentoring some of your newer nursing colleagues. One day, you will also become a mentor to those entering the nurse practitioner (NP) profession. What type of mentor will you be? What characteristics will you possess? Will they be some of the same characteristics you are searching for in a mentor yourself?

This chapter expands on the importance of mentoring others. Reasons why NPs rely so much on these relationships are discussed. Mentoring is described as our particular way to reshape the future of our discipline.

In this chapter, you will learn:

1. Why you should be a mentor
2. What type of mentor you should be

ME — A MENTOR?

It is never too early to start thinking about becoming a mentor. Let me explain why. **You have chosen to become part of a profession that relies heavily on preceptors and mentors.**

I chose to group these two functions together for the last part of this discussion, as they often overlap.

At the time of this writing, no formal means of reimbursement for preceptors exists. They receive only the recognition for having volunteered to be a preceptor, which is given at the time of NP recertification. Some schools also offer adjunct status, which gives the preceptor access to the library and other resources. With the need for NPs predicted to rise, there will also be an increased need for qualified preceptors. This factor and others, such as higher patient loads, more seriously ill patients, economic factors, and the responsibility of working with a student, may lead to an insufficient number of NPs volunteering to serve as preceptors. This is and likely will continue to be a factor affecting NP education.

To me, good mentors are knowledgeable. They are competent. They are confident, yet modest. They are approachable and available. They will give advice when asked, but will listen when nothing is asked for. They are open and nonjudgmental. They are honest and trustworthy. They are role models.

=== *FAST FACTS in a NUTSHELL*

- The NP profession relies heavily on mentors.
- With the need for NPs predicted to rise, there will also be an increased need for qualified preceptors.

WHY SHOULD I BE A MENTOR?

I hope you all will serve as mentors and, more formally, as preceptors, for future NP students and new NPs. In 2010, I responded to an editorial written on this important topic, stating that, for me, precepting and mentoring NP students has been and always will be a part of my professional responsibilities (Aktan, 2010). It is an honor to be asked to mentor or precept future colleagues.

So why should you be a mentor? You will get a sense of satisfaction out of helping those who look to you for guidance. This is how you will begin to participate in reshaping the future of our discipline. You will reap the benefits, as well. When we become involved in facilitating our colleagues' effective transition to the NP role, we are helping to strengthen the field, both now and in the future.

How can you start this process? You probably already have. Novice nurses have looked to you for advice. They have gotten to know you and respect you. Once they hear you are enrolled in an NP program or are considering becoming an NP, they will come to you.

As previously discussed, increasingly nurses are being encouraged to go to graduate school sooner than they were ever before. They have lots of questions and will look to those who have already begun the journey. Share what you have learned and provide encouragement. Has not someone done this for you?

FAST FACTS in a NUTSHELL

- By becoming a mentor you will have the opportunity to reshape the future of our discipline.
- Share what you have learned and provide encouragement.

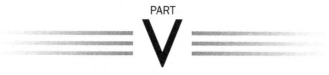

PART

V

Attaining Your Certification and Licensure

9

Who? What? Where?

Certification is an essential part of nurse practitioner (NP) practice. Regulations vary from state to state but, in general, you need to obtain certification to manage your own patients. It is critical to review the certification requirements of potential employers. After graduation, your school will forward your eligibility to sit for certification examinations on your request. It is then time to get started!

This chapter presents the certification options available for NPs in the various specialty areas in an unbiased format, including criteria for eligibility and guidelines for registration. Several organizations offer NP certification. These are explored and explained.

In this chapter, you will learn:

1. Recommendations for certification
2. Organizations that certify NPs
3. How to apply for certification

TYPES OF NURSE PRACTITIONER CERTIFICATIONS AVAILABLE

A variety of organizations offer NP certification. You must carefully review all options within your area of expertise. The Internet offers a wealth of information. Most importantly, talk to experts in the field. This is the best way to consider the types of NP certifications available.

The American Academy of Nurse Practitioners (AANP) and the American Nurses Credentialing Center (ANCC) are the two primary national certifying bodies for NPs. The AANP (http://aanp.org) currently offers three specialty certifications (see Table 9.1). The ANCC has a nationally recognized program with 10 different certifications for NPs (www.nursecredentialing.org/Certification). These are listed in Table 9.2. Other organizations that offer additional NP certifications are referenced in Table 9.3.

TABLE 9.1 AANP Specialty Certifications

Adult–Gerontology
Adult (to be retired 2017)
Gerontological (retired 2012)
Family

TABLE 9.2 ANCC Specialty Certifications

Acute Care
Adult
Adult–Gerontology Acute Care
Adult–Gerontology Primary Care
Family
Gerontological
Pediatric
Adult Psychiatric/Mental Health
Psychiatric/Mental Health
Advanced Diabetes Management (retired)
School (retired)
Emergency

TABLE 9.3 Sources of Additional Nurse Practitioner Certifications
American Association of Critical Care Nurses (http://www.aacn.org/wd/certifications/content/ccrnlanding.pcms?menu=certification)
National Certification Corporation for the Obstetric, Gynecological, and Neonatal Nursing Specialties (www.nccwebsite.org)
Pediatric Nursing Certification Board (www.pncb.org)

The National Certification Corporation (NCC) is a not-for-profit organization that provides a national credentialing program for nurses and other licensed health care personnel. This organization provides the *registered nurse, certified* (RNC) credential as a women's health or neonatal nurse practitioner. Information can be found on the organization's website (www.nccwebsite.org). Once you have carefully explored the types of NP certification available, you will be ready to evaluate the criteria for eligibility and, then, the process for registration.

═══════════════════════════*FAST FACTS in a NUTSHELL*

AANP and AACN are the two primary national organizations that certify NPs.

CRITERIA FOR ELIGIBILITY AND REGISTRATION

You must carefully review and understand the criteria for certification eligibility and registration guidelines for certification. I recommend you do so before selecting a graduate program to be sure you will be eligible for the certification you are interested in obtaining. You will then need to stay current about these guidelines as you complete your requirements and prepare to register for taking the certification examination. The criteria for eligibility and guidelines for registration, as well as applications, can be found and downloaded at the websites provided in Table 9.3.

My opinion, based on my experiences, is that national certification is important and, in most cases, essential. It demonstrates to potential and current employers, as well as to colleagues, patients, and their families, that the NP is competent in his or her specialty area.

Some practitioners support attaining more than one certification, possibly all those offered in your specialty area. I am not certain this is a critical element for success. It is, however, something to consider based on your own personal and professional career goals.

I am ANCC certified. At the time I graduated, this option was recommended to me by my mentors and colleagues in the field. I have worked with many AANP-certified colleagues throughout the years and believe this alternate certification to be equally acceptable. My recommendation is to talk to your preceptors, mentors, other NPs in your specialty area, and potential future employers to ascertain their preferred certifying agency.

FAST FACTS in a NUTSHELL

- It is up to you to carefully review and understand the criteria for NP certification eligibility and registration.
- My opinion, based on my experiences, is that national certification is important and, in most cases, essential.

10

Passing

Be realistic. Nothing presented in this book will mean much to you unless you can be successful on your certification examination. Think back to your nursing boards. Do you ever want to do that again? Not likely. Therefore, to save your money and your sanity, you need to remain focused on passing—the first time. There are a few key strategies for doing so.

This chapter presents recommendations for passing certification exams. The major nurse practitioner (NP) review courses are also compared. Concepts such as familiarizing yourself with test-taking strategies and policies related to taking your certification exam on the computer should also be considered.

In this chapter, you will learn:

1. Ways to be certain you are successful on your certification examination
2. The test preparation resources available

HOW TO PASS—THE FIRST TIME

There are several ways to facilitate the successful completion of certification examinations. Overall, my recommendation is to **prepare for NP certification by taking practice tests that contain exam-format questions, and studying and understanding the accompanying rationales.** The more questions, the better.

You can do so in a variety of ways. Options include review books, flashcards, websites, apps and computer programs, and, possibly, registering for and participating in a review course. It is important that the materials you use to prepare coincide with the exam you plan to take (e.g., family guides for the family exam). Asking your preceptors or mentors who have successfully passed the certification exam you intend to take how they prepared would be an excellent way to start.

===================*FAST FACTS in a NUTSHELL*

> The more test questions you practice taking and rationales you understand, the higher the likelihood of success.

REVIEW COURSES

For me, a review course was the best way to identify my weaknesses and formulate a plan for study. I cannot stress these two factors enough. You must have a plan.

Review courses incorporate the main concepts expected to appear on a certification examination, as they are often based on the most recent test questions. Usually, useful materials are included in the cost of the course. These items alone are often worth the expense of the entire course.

Although not everyone may need or want to spend money on a review course, you will need to purchase (or borrow) some formalized review materials. I took a course, and also bought and borrowed books.

I was also part of one of the last groups to take the American Nurses Credentialing Center (ANCC) family nurse practitioner (FNP) boards as a pencil-and-paper examination.

Therefore, I did not need to review computerized exam materials. Today, this is the only means of testing offered, so you also must familiarize yourself with computerized testing strategies and policies related to your certification exam—especially if you do not consider yourself tech savvy! *Do not* allow yourself to be distracted from the content of the questions because you are uncomfortable with the means of testing. Know how the computer-based examination is administered and the types of items to expect. You will be anxious enough about mastering the content without worrying about the technical aspects of test taking!

A straightforward, seemingly nonbiased comparison of the major NP review courses is available from the NP Central website (www.npcentral.net/ce/review.shtml). The review courses described there are listed in Table 10.1.

I chose a particular review course for two reasons. One was there was a money-back guarantee if I did not pass (which I did!). The other was that I met the course leader at a conference, and she explained how she uses hands-on learning techniques as a teaching strategy, so that attendees do not just sit all day listening to lectures. Instead, she has them get up and participate. I know that I am a visual learner, so this type of preparation made sense for me. In fact, I still use strategies I learned during this experience to remember important practice tips today. Yet, interactive teaching–learning strategies are not right for everyone. Think about the type of learner you are and consider this while researching and reviewing the various types of programs available.

Explore the various review courses available and ask those who have participated for their feedback. I have heard positive feedback from colleagues about all of the major

TABLE 10.1 Nurse Practitioner Review Courses and Providers

Advanced Practice Education Associates (APEA)

Fitzgerald Health Education Associates NP Certification Exam Review

Marye Dorsey Kellermann's Necessary NP Review

review programs available. Their individual websites provide a wealth of information but, as usual, the "real scoop" comes directly from those who have taken the various courses (and passed). This is usually the best bet to guide you in the right direction.

════════════════════════ FAST FACTS in a NUTSHELL

- Identify your weaknesses and formulate a plan for study.
- Review courses incorporate the main concepts expected to appear on a certification examination.
- A nonbiased comparison of the major NP review courses is available at http://www.npcentral.net/ce/review.shtml.
- The "real scoop" comes directly from those who have taken the various courses (and passed).

DEVELOPING A STUDY PLAN

Once you have selected your materials, develop a plan for study. There is a tremendous amount of information to review and remember. This is *not* a task that can be allotted to a couple of days or weekends—and certainly not something to be left until the night before. The process of preparation requires constant, consistent focus. It requires time, and energy.

I do not recommend waiting too long after graduation to begin your exam preparations. In fact, you should register to take the exam as soon as possible. Often several weeks to months are spent simply getting all of your "ducks in order" to be eligible. This should be sufficient time to prepare. If too much time elapses, your recall of valuable knowledge may start to fade.

I took a few weeks off from work right before my exam. I developed and adhered to a schedule for study. This is what worked best for me. My plan was based on pretesting and results from a review course that helped me identify the areas on which I needed to focus. Everyone has strengths and weaknesses. If you are scoring well on certain topics, then move on to test areas where you are not scoring quite so high.

Finally, think about this: How did you prepare for your nursing boards? Did you study alone or in groups? Did you prepare using books or other testing materials? Did you participate in a review course? What additional resources were helpful for you? Most importantly, were you successful? This is likely to be the most influential factor in your decision on where to go from here.

TEST YOURSELF

Answer the following true/false questions to see what you learned in this chapter:

1. I must enroll in a review course to pass my certification exam.
2. I can borrow a colleague's FNP review materials to study for the adult–gerontology nurse practitioner exam.
3. I am computer savvy, so I do not need to review computerized test-taking strategies.
4. There is no reason why I should not be able to cram the weekend before the test.
5. If I study my notes from my classes, I will be adequately prepared.

Of course, the simple answer to all of these questions is *false*. It is not mandatory that you take a review course, although most experts in the field recommend it. You must, however, prepare using materials developed for the specialty examination that you intend to take. It is highly recommended that you become competent in all test-taking strategies, particularly those for computer-based examinations. It is not likely that cramming the weekend before the test will be adequate preparation. Although course notes may be helpful, materials that have been specifically developed for the exams (books, flashcards, apps, computer programs, and *lots of questions*) are your best bets for success.

- Preparing for your NP certification examination requires constant, consistent focus, time, and energy.
- Register to take the exam as soon as possible.

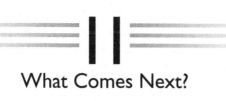

What Comes Next?

The next step in preparing for nurse practitioner (NP) practice is licensure. Although this process varies from state to state, it is important to understand basic guidelines and principles related to NP licensure. As usual, asking your mentors, current employers, or potential employers which licenses you will be required to obtain is a prudent way to begin.

This chapter discusses the various licenses an NP will consider applying for and the importance of each. Factors such as cost, reimbursement, and protection of your NP license are discussed.

In this chapter, you will learn:

1. A basic overview of the types of licenses for which NPs are eligible to apply
2. Recommendations regarding licensure
3. Strategies for obtaining and protecting your NP license

THE TYPES OF LICENSES A NURSE PRACTITIONER WILL NEED

Once you successfully pass your certification examination, you will be eligible to apply for state licensure. You will still maintain your current nursing (RN) license, but, in addition, you will be required to apply for the NP license. This will allow you to practice according to your individual state guidelines. It will also allow you to prescribe in most states. To bill for services, you will need to obtain a national provider identification (NPI) number.

In the state where I practice, a controlled dangerous substance (CDS) license is required in order to prescribe controlled substances. This qualifies the provider to obtain a Drug Enforcement Administration (DEA) number. These two items permit you to prescribe controlled substances legally. This process may vary slightly from state to state.

This process continues to change and evolve—seemingly by the minute. This is why it is important to stay current on the latest guidelines. Reading professional journals, attending NP conferences, and staying in touch with professional colleagues are some of the ways to stay informed. Joining your professional organizations is another way to keep current on the latest guidelines for licensure.

The best place to start the NP licensure process is with your state board of nursing. Usually, all pertinent information is available right on its website. Relevant contact information should also be provided there in the event you require additional clarification.

=== *FAST FACTS in a NUTSHELL*

NPs must maintain both RN and NP licenses. They may also apply for a CDS license, and DEA and NPI numbers.

THE PROCESS OF LICENSURE

Obtaining—and maintaining—all of these licenses can be expensive, so you need to plan for it. The cost of licensure and license renewals is something that you may be able to successfully negotiate into your employment contract (see Chapter 18 for more details).

Again, begin the process by checking the website of your state board of nursing, where you can find application guidelines, fees, and contact information. In most cases, you can apply online. Once you are employed, other NPs or office personnel may be able to assist you in determining what is needed at your practice site(s) and what you need to do to get started.

Ask mentors and employers which licenses you are expected to maintain. As a general rule, you should apply for and maintain every license for which you are eligible. This way, no matter how the rules change, you will always have the necessary licenses. Yet, this could become expensive and might not be necessary for all NPs. For example, if your practice site treats clients with a history of substance abuse and maintains a policy that no controlled substances are prescribed, it may not be necessary for you to possess a CDS license and maintain your DEA number. Only you can decide, but you should think about it carefully.

Suppose you decide you do need to apply for a CDS license and a DEA number. The CDS is usually less than a hundred dollars; however, the DEA cost more than seven hundred dollars to renew in 2013. The NPI number application is free—for now! Of course, you will also be expected to maintain your state nursing (RN) license, as well as apply for your state advanced practicing nursing (NP) license. The cost of applying for these licenses may vary greatly from state to state, but most likely it will require several hundred dollars to obtain and slightly less to maintain each of these.

========================*FAST FACTS in a NUTSHELL*

Your state board of nursing website should provide you with most of the information necessary to become licensed as an NP.

MAINTAINING AND PROTECTING YOUR NURSE PRACTITIONER LICENSE

Finally, you need to maintain your professional NP license. Just as with your nursing license, your NP license can be suspended or revoked for a variety of reasons. Of course, malpractice suits, in which you may be found to have practiced outside of standards or guidelines, put your NP license in jeopardy.

Chapter 20 provides a wealth of information about protection from lawsuits. This, in turn, helps protect your license. Review it carefully. Other situations, such as criminal behavior or substance abuse violations, could also result in a permanent or temporary loss of licensure. It is ultimately your responsibility to stay current with regulations and to follow the appropriate guidelines for license renewal.

In addition, always notify the state board of nursing, any other relevant licensing boards, and your certifying body if there are name or other changes in your contact information, just as you would with your RN license. As mentioned, you are responsible for keeping your licenses current and complying with all regulations. By maintaining membership in professional organizations and attending conferences, this should not be difficult to do.

═══════════════════════*FAST FACTS in a NUTSHELL*

- Professional malpractice, criminal behavior, or substance abuse violations can result in permanent or temporary loss of licensure.
- Just as with your RN license, you need to maintain and protect your NP license.

PART

VI

Surviving and Thriving:
Your First Year in Practice

12

First Job

This chapter guides the reader through various ways to obtain a position as a nurse practitioner (NP)—the right position for you—and some pitfalls to avoid. It also provides an in-depth analysis of issues a new NP is likely to encounter on the job and how to best manage them.

After landing your ideal position, you will be faced with a number of issues, particularly when first assuming the role of a novice practitioner. One of these is the job description itself, which may be difficult to understand from both the nursing perspective and that of other health care professionals with whom NPs work. It is important to understand factors that may alleviate these difficulties, which are described in this chapter.

In this chapter, you will learn:

1. How to identify and select your first NP position
2. What to look for in an NP position
3. What to avoid in an NP position

HOW TO BECOME EMPLOYED AS A NURSE PRACTITIONER

Selecting your first position as an NP may present challenges. How should you begin? Where should you look? What should you avoid?

First, of course, you need to determine where positions are available. Online search engines for job listings are likely the best place to start. **Hospitals and other large institutions post open positions on their own websites and through their human resources departments.** However, this is only the beginning.

By now, you have begun the process of networking. You have developed a network of contacts through your work as a nurse. You have contacts through your school and faculty. You have contacts through clinical sites and preceptors. You have contacts with your classmates and your mentors. Ask! The best NP positions available may not always be posted.

Here is an additional strategy. When I was considering a job change, I compiled a list of all the primary/urgent care centers in my geographical area where I would consider working. I then prepared a cover letter describing my ideal position and the characteristics I possessed that would contribute to a successful practice. I attached my curriculum vitae and mailed it to the lead physician in the practices I had identified, approximately 30 in all.

Remember, these were "cold calls" in the sense that none had posted vacant positions. I received several calls and went on three or four interviews. Most did not turn out to be what I was looking for. One did. I have been with this practice for more than 15 years. See what time, effort, and patience can do?

What unique strategy can you devise to successfully promote yourself and land your ideal NP position?

- Posted NP positions are only the beginning. Network and think "outside the box!"
- Use the network you have created through your colleagues, classmates, faculty members, preceptors, and mentors.

POTENTIAL PITFALLS

It may be tempting to remain at your current place of employment for your first NP position. You already know the ropes, so to speak. You know the patients, you know the employees, and you know "the system."

You should, however, consider choosing a practice site different from the site you worked in as a nurse. Colleagues who have worked closely with you as a registered nurse (RN) may have difficulty in comprehending or acknowledging your NP role. This does not mean you should not stay within the same institution—possibly you would be at ease with just a different setting within the organization. Consider the following scenario and answer the question at the end, which addresses this important point.

Julie, a seasoned emergency room nurse, recently began a new job as an NP. She was thrilled to be offered a position in the same emergency department in which she has worked for more than 10 years. Here, she will be working closely with Scott, another NP, who was one of her preceptors and has also been an important mentor to her.

All has been going well, and Julie is thriving in the new position. One busy morning, Julie is evaluating a pediatric patient who fell off his bicycle and hit his head. His mother is concerned that he may have lost consciousness. While she is evaluating the patient, Sharon, Julie's former nurse manager, who is also a friend, pulls her aside.

Sharon tells Julie that Dr. Phillips is furious; he ordered a urinalysis and blood glucose level on his patient and it has not yet been completed. Sharon asks Julie to pitch in and help out. Put yourself in Julie's shoes. What should you do?

1. Ignore Sharon.
2. Ask Scott to address Sharon.
3. Get the urinalysis and blood glucose level.
4. Quit.
5. Tell Sharon that although you are a team player and do not mind helping out, these are the responsibilities of the nurse. Now you must focus on your NP role, as you manage a complex clinical patient.

Correct answer: 5.
In evaluating the possible answers, consider the following:

1. Ignoring a manager is never a good option, even if you do not report to him or her.
2. If Scott were still Julie's preceptor, this option might be appropriate. However, Scott and Julie now have a different relationship—they are colleagues. Therefore, it is not appropriate to ask Scott to address Sharon.
3. Although agreeing to help out may be a quick way to address the situation, it does not set a good precedent. Occasionally, it may be appropriate for the NP to take on nursing responsibilities to help out, but you have to be careful. This should never distract you from patients you are responsible for managing.
4. If this sort of behavior continues, it may be time to consider other positions. However, I certainly do not advocate quitting at this time.
5. Option five is the best answer. Allowing yourself to be distracted from a complex clinical case can negatively affect patient outcomes. Your colleagues need to understand your new role.

This example highlights why remaining in a situation where colleagues could confuse your new NP role with your previous nursing role may not be the best choice. However, with the right approach and support from the start, you may be able to successfully transition to your new role in the same setting.

You are now ready for the next step. The remaining chapters in Part VI will prepare you to transition into your new NP role, and thrive while doing so.

FAST FACTS in a NUTSHELL

- Consider changing your practice site from a previous setting where you have worked as a nurse.
- With the right approach, however, you may be able to successfully remain in the same setting.

12. FIRST JOB

13

Role Transition

Transitioning from the role of the registered nurse (RN) to the role of the nurse practitioner (NP) is a process that takes time and effort. At times, it may seem difficult. Identifying some key players in the successful transition is recommended. It is imperative that, right from the beginning, the NP role be established and clarified. You should make your new role understood and be certain your collaborating physician does so as well.

This chapter presents guidelines for successfully transitioning into the NP role. Ways to avoid practicing outside of the NP role are described. Other ideas that promote positive role transition are also provided.

In this chapter, you will learn:

1. How to establish and adhere to the NP role
2. How to avoid practicing outside of the role
3. Suggestions for surviving the transition

DEFINING THE NP ROLE

To effectively transition, from day one, the NP role must be clearly defined. The role must be understood by the NP *and* by those alongside whom he or she works. Key players in the successful transition include, but are not limited to, physicians and administrators, other NPs, nurses, medical and nursing assistants, other technicians (e.g., radiology), managerial personnel, and support staff. Guidelines to ensure that the NP does not function, and is not expected to function, as a sort of glorified nurse must be established. That is not the intention of the NP role. In many practice settings, NPs function in the same or a similar way as our physician colleagues. Yet, office staff and other personnel may have difficulty accepting this new hierarchy.

Often, the NP is seen as functioning somewhere in between the physician and other nurses. Right from the start, I recommend differentiating oneself as an independent practitioner with the knowledge and skills to contribute to the organization or practice at a higher level than an RN. Furthermore, I do not support the use of a term commonly seen in the literature to describe the NP role—"physician extender." If you examine the history of the NP role, this is not who we are or who we set out to be.

NPs are independent practitioners with their own clearly defined scope of practice. Any NP textbook will tell you this. You learned this in your first NP course. If you retain any concept contained in this book, let it be this: *You are no extender*—to a physician or anyone else for that matter. You worked too hard to settle for this title!

The transition process may be easier when the practice or institution has previously employed NPs. Here, all members of the multidisciplinary team may have been exposed to the roles and responsibilities of the NP. But this is not always so. How the NP who came before you functioned within the role could affect the expectations of others. Again, you need to be clear as to what *your* role will include.

═══════════════════════════ FAST FACTS in a NUTSHELL

- To effectively transition into the NP role, it must be clearly defined from day one.
- NPs are independent practitioners with their own clearly defined scope of practice.

HOW WILL YOU BEGIN TO DEFINE YOUR NEW ROLE?

What will be your role in the practice or institution? Get it in writing! Your collaborative agreement is an acceptable place to start defining your role (see Chapter 22 for more information). Yet, even a clearly written definition of the role will not entirely address some potential problems related to role transition. That is why I recommend that you avoid practicing outside the role.

This being said, no matter how many credentials we have after our names, we are still nurses. When I am practicing as an NP and see a patient standing with a cup of urine in his or her hand, I take the cup from the patient and dip it for urinalysis. It is not often that I see a doctor do the same. This is where the gray area persists in the NP role. Let me be clear: I have no problem dipping a cup of urine. The problem I have is that I have accepted the legal and ethical responsibility for managing patients. If I am distracted from my work by doing something that a nurse or another member of the health care team can perform within his or her job description, my focus has shifted from the role of the NP to that of the nurse. As an experienced NP, I know that this may be acceptable at times, but it could lead to trouble for a novice NP.

===========================*FAST FACTS in a NUTSHELL*

> Your collaborative agreement is an acceptable place to start defining your role.

YOUR OWN UNIQUE IDENTITY AND PHILOSOPHY

So what should you do? This is another area in which you need to make some decisions for yourself. I am not advocating that NPs get up on their high horses, refusing to be team players or to help out when help is needed. What I am recommending is that **your role be clear.** Clear to you. Clear to your collaborating physician. Clear to other colleagues and employees. Clear to your patients.

For instance, if your patients see you taking vital signs, and this is something they have always seen done by the nurse and never by the physician, do you see how this may interfere with patients' acceptance of the NP role and, more specifically, your role in assuming a leadership position in managing their care? Think about it. Decide what is right for you.

═══════════════════════════ *FAST FACTS in a NUTSHELL*

Establish your own identity and philosophy in accordance with your institutional or practice policies and state guidelines.

BECOME AN EFFECTIVE DELEGATOR—AGAIN!

There is one more important aspect to ensuring a proper transition into the new NP role—effective delegation. As nurses, we have to delegate all the time. Some nurses are, of course, better at this than others. I have never been good at delegating; it is a concept that I still struggle with today. Yet, in our current challenged health care system, we are caring for increasingly complex patients. We rely on licensed assistive personnel to help us to meet the demands placed on us. To effectively manage their clients' care, nurses need to delegate.

As a novice NP, you will have to learn how to delegate all over again. This may be difficult to some because, at times, it is other nurses to whom you are delegating. How do you feel about this? It may be harder than you think. Consider the following scenario as you reflect on the concept of NP delegation:

Melissa, a new pediatric nurse practitioner (PNP), has been transitioning into her role at a thriving pediatric practice. As stipulated in her contract, after 6 months of employment, Melissa is to work independently every other Saturday morning to manage the practice's sick visits. Overall, Melissa has been managing this new responsibility well.

One busy Saturday morning during cough and cold season, the medical assistant calls in sick. Melissa has already seen 12 patients in the first 2 hours. The receptionist keeps transferring calls with clinical questions back to the nurses' station, and the nurse, Sarah, is answering them.

Because she is on the phone, Sarah is not bringing patients into the rooms in a timely fashion. In fact, she has stopped bringing them in at all. She has also decided that she will no longer be taking the patients' vital signs because she is "too busy." Sarah has also already interrupted Melissa several times with clinical questions related to the phone calls from parents.

Put yourself in Melissa's place. What should you do?

1. Bring the patients into the room and take the vitals yourself.
2. Reprimand the receptionist for transferring the calls and Sarah for answering them.
3. Ask the receptionist to take messages on all phone calls that are not emergencies. Take Sarah aside and tell her that even though it is her usual responsibility to triage phone calls, today's situation requires her to fulfill a different role. She is to bring in patients and take their vital signs so that you can be more effective in managing them. Together you will return phone calls after patient care is completed.

Correct answer: 3.
In evaluating the possible answers, consider the following:

1. Assuming nursing responsibilities yourself will not help you manage the patient flow. It can also distract you from patient management, which is your role in this scenario.
2. Reprimanding anyone will not likely help the situation. In addition, it may make the other employees resent working with you.

3. Coming up with a plan and delegating responsibilities is the most effective way to manage this situation.

=== *FAST FACTS in a NUTSHELL*

Effective delegation is an important aspect of the NP role.

BE CREATIVE

I have one additional "outside the box" suggestion for surviving your first year of NP practice: **participate in a medical mission.** An excellent time to participate in this life-changing endeavor would be during graduate school. I understand this option may not be always practical because of academic and other commitments. So, an alternate time to explore this facet of your ongoing education might be just before you begin your first NP position.

Early in my last semester as a family nurse practitioner (FNP) student, one of my teachers and mentors began to talk about Puerto Eten, a town in her native Peru. Two years prior, the town had been devastated by a flood and more than 200 families had been living in tents ever since—with no access to health care. She was planning a trip and asked others who might want to accompany her to apply to join this mission. I immediately applied and was selected along with other NP and nursing students.

We arrived with our penlights, stethoscopes, and blood pressure cuffs; some boxes of medications; urine dip sticks; and a glucometer. We used what we had. We had our eyes, our ears, our hands, and our instincts. What we did not have was an ECG machine, a laboratory, or an x-ray machine. We had no other means of diagnostic testing. This is how you can and will take your skills to the next level—the NP level.

I remember being led to a tiny, dark, withering tent by a nervous new father who spoke no English in order for me to examine his wife and new baby. As a nurse, I had performed a postpartum and neonatal assessments hundreds of times before. Yet, this time was different. I had no tools. No scale for daily weights. No means to measure bilirubin. No life-saving vaccines to administer.

I performed a postpartum evaluation using only the light shining through a flap in the tent. I carried the baby out in the sunlight to check its color. I continued through every newborn assessment parameter I could think of that did not require an instrument. This experience opened my eyes to how dependent I had become on technology.

I did have tools. I had my senses. I had my knowledge. I had my experience. I am a more effective practitioner today because of the time I spent on this mission. Think about it. There will always be jobs; there may not always be an opportunity for adventure combined with learning.

═══════════════════════*FAST FACTS in a NUTSHELL*

Participate in innovative opportunities to take your skills to the NP level.

14

Friends and Enemies

In any job, it is critical to identify those who will help you effectively transition into your new role. Coworkers and other colleagues can provide insight based on their own knowledge and experience in a particular setting. Make it your business to find friends and avoid enemies.

The chapter clarifies ways to seek out key players who will help you as a new nurse practitioner (NP), your "friends," so to speak. Ways to avoid making "enemies," or those who may interfere with your effective role transition, are discussed. The rationales for these important relationships are also provided.

In this chapter, you will learn:

1. To identify those who will help you effectively transition into the NP role
2. To avoid those who will not help you transition
3. The reasons why this is important to a new NP

FINDING FRIENDS AND AVOIDING ENEMIES

Who will be your friend as a new NP? Well, anyone can be your friend. You need friends right now. You need lots of them. What you do not need are enemies. You do not need a jealous colleague or a difficult administrator. You need support. You need patience. If you are supportive and patient, it is likely you will be treated this way in return.

Of course, life has taught me that this is not always so. I am not naïve nor am I asking you to be. You can be easy to work with and still get stuck with difficult coworkers.

Physicians and other NPs who will be patient, answer questions, and share their own interesting cases as learning experiences are your friends. Nurses and other staff members who will show you how the practice or institution runs and the best ways to manage routines are also your friends. An x-ray technician or another professional with years of experience is another valuable friend. Although interpreting a test is not in his or her job description, an experienced technician can be an invaluable resource in guiding you in the right direction during your first few months.

Often an office manager, administrator, or receptionist can be an important friend early in your NP practice. They usually know the patients and their families. They know the other employees. They may even know the managers or receptionists in other offices. They know how to get an important diagnostic test precertified, promptly. They know how to obtain an urgent appointment for your patient with a specialist when there is a 3-month waiting list. Although you are an experienced nurse with knowledge, skills, and a drive to succeed, you probably do not yet know many of these critical facets of NP practice.

You will, in time. But right now your energy must be expended on collecting a thorough history, performing a comprehensive physical examination, diagnosing, and managing—not trying to obtain emergency department room reports or the results of your patient's mammogram. Individuals who can help you with these sorts of tasks are your allies. Make them your friends and keep it that way. Buy them a cup of coffee when you buy yourself one. It will be well worth it.

- Physicians, other NPs, and other colleagues who are patient and supportive are invaluable resources for the new NP.
- An office manager, administrator, or receptionist can also be an important friend early in your NP practice.

Consider the following scenario and answer the question at the end to see what you have learned in this chapter.

Mary is a newly licensed family nurse practitioner (FNP). She graduated in the top of her class and has more than 15 years of hospital experience. Mary accepted a position in a busy urgent care center and is ready to practice. During her first few weeks, Mary struggled with grasping the basic patient flow of the center, while providing care for a large number of patients, most of whom are seen on a walk-in basis.

Beth, a nonpracticing RN, is the office manager. Although ultimately responsible for nonmedical staff, Beth frequently comes into the busy clinical area and criticizes the flow of patient care. Usually Beth is polite toward Mary. However, a month into the job, Beth tells Mary that she is not seeing patients quickly enough. She says so in a loud, confrontational tone and does so in front of all of the other clinical employees. How should Mary best respond?

1. Mary should ignore her.
2. Mary should increase her pace and see patients more quickly.
3. Mary should raise her voice louder than Beth in the clinical area, responding that she is the NP and how dare Beth speak to her this way.
4. Mary should report Beth to her collaborating physician.
5. Mary should calmly ask to speak with Beth in private. Clearly and firmly Mary should ask Beth not to confront her in this way, especially in front of other employees. Mary should ask Beth to discuss future concerns with her

directly or with her collaborating physician, as that is the person to whom Mary reports.

Correct answer: 5
In evaluating the possible answers, consider the following:

1. Although ignoring Beth may be an effective strategy temporarily, this option does not address her inappropriate approach.
2. Although it may be necessary, in time, for Mary to increase the pace at which she sees patients, it is not Beth's role to address this with Mary, as an NP should not report to an office manager.
3. Although it may be tempting to confront Beth on the spot, arguing with her will not make this situation any better. In fact, it could make the situation worse.
4. If this sort of behavior continues, it may be necessary to discuss the situation with Beth's supervisor or someone else in authority. This is not, however, the best initial strategy if the situation can be resolved between them.
5. Common sense would suggest that diffusing the conflict is a more effective initial approach to the problem. By working together, Mary and Beth could come up with a way to address this issue in a more professional way.

Beth could easily become an enemy, but this need not happen. She could also become a friend (believe it or not). Beth may have felt threatened initially by Mary's new role at the center and may have viewed this confrontation as a way to test the waters. It is highly possible the Mary has passed Beth's "test" and a mutually respectful work environment can be created between them.

So let's review: Who are your friends? Only you know the answer. Identify your weaknesses. Anyone who can help you overcome them is a friend.

EXAMPLE: DR. SMITH

Here is a personal example that illustrates why it is so important to make friends as a new NP. Cardiology has always been one of my shortcomings. ST-wave elevations give me chest pain! Early on, I found a friend, Dr. Smith, who is an extremely bright, pleasant, patient cardiologist. Soon after meeting him I realized that he, or another partner from his group, would always promptly return my phone calls.

I have referred hundreds of patients to him for cardiac workups over the years. In turn, I can call him when concerned about a patient, and he will get right back to me. Dr. Smith always ensures that he, or another specialist in his group, is available for patients needing timely cardiac evaluations.

Over time, I have become more comfortable in determining which patients with cardiac symptoms or abnormal ECG findings needed immediate attention. Dr. Smith was a friend to me as a novice NP. He is still a friend today. This is an example of why finding and keeping friends is a critical element of early NP practice.

FAST FACTS in a NUTSHELL

Any colleague who can help you overcome some of your shortcomings is a friend.

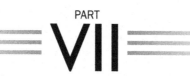

PART

VII

Administrative Issues

15

Bureaucracy

The nurse practitioner (NP) is faced with a variety of bureaucratic issues that may affect his or her practice. Therefore, the NP must understand the hierarchy of the practice or institution. It is equally important that other employees be aware of the levels of hierarchy, and where the NP fits within them.

This chapter presents the most common issues related to the bureaucracy of a practice or institution that challenge NP practice. How the institution's hierarchy affects the NP's role is discussed. Related pitfalls, as well as recommendations for preventing or managing them, also are discussed.

In this chapter, you will learn:

1. Ways to prevent issues that can adversely affect NP practice
2. How NPs fit into the hierarchy and proper reporting procedures
3. Issues to consider in establishing an independent NP practice

AVOIDING BUREAUCRATIC TRAPS

The bureaucracy of a practice or institution can be as challenging as many of the complex clinical cases facing a new

NP. As in many other professions, the NP must often deal with reams of red tape. This need not be the case! Red tape may be minimized if planned for and addressed early in the transition into the new NP role.

An unclear chain of command is one of the most complex bureaucratic traps into which a new NP can fall. Address the issue right from the start. The best time would be during contract negotiations. (The importance of contracts is addressed in Chapter 18.) At this point, you should understand that from day one the NP must be completely clear as to about whom he or she is expected to report to. As previously discussed, this should be put in writing.

In many practices, some nurses, assistants, and support staff report to an office administrator. In most instances, this is *not* an appropriate supervisor for the professional NP. More appropriately, an NP should report directly to his or her collaborating physician or the owner of a practice, a medical director, a lead NP, or the chief nursing administrator or officer of an institution. This list is, of course, not inclusive. Other examples of appropriate peers or colleagues can also be considered. Often, this decision depends on the policy of the institution or practice.

FAST FACTS in a NUTSHELL

Appropriate professionals to whom the NP may report are the collaborating physician or the owner of a practice, a medical director, a lead NP, or the chief nursing administrator or officer of the institution.

AVOIDING ROLE CONFLICTS

If the NP or others are uncertain as to whom the NP reports, problems will probably develop. Consider the following scenario and answer the questions at the end to see what you have learned.

Celeste, an adult–gerontology nurse practitioner (AGNP), has been hired by the medical department of a large urban hospital. She is to assist the endocrinology unit in managing the overwhelming aspects of care related to newly diagnosed clients with type 2 diabetes. Celeste assumes that she will report to the medical department, as members of this department had interviewed and hired her.

Early on, responsibilities are delegated to Celeste by Dr. Schwartz, the institution's chief of endocrinology. Celeste determines this to be consistent with what she had learned was appropriate to the NP role. She performs her duties within the NP scope of practice. Dr. Schwartz is pleased with her contributions to the department. He provides Celeste with a highly positive performance evaluation after her first 3 months.

Robert, the director of nursing, has recently been faced with severe budget cuts. He has been asked to reduce staffing at all levels without reduction in care. As a result, Robert transferred two diabetes educators to another institution within the same health care system. Now, he needs to consider how to ensure that patient care is not affected by this decision.

According to the organizational chart, NPs report directly to the nursing department. Therefore, Robert decides to delegate aspects of the educators' previous responsibilities directly to Celeste. He does not discuss this decision with Dr. Schwartz or anyone else from the medical department.

Upon being made aware of these new responsibilities, Celeste becomes concerned. Not only is she juggling a full workload of NP responsibilities, she is now faced with a number of new, time-consuming activities that members of the nursing staff are more than qualified to perform. Celeste decides that she is a team player. She does not want to complain to Dr. Schwartz. Therefore, she assumes the additional duties.

At first, Celeste is able to manage her increased workload, even though at times she must stay late and come in early. She is not paid for overtime. But Celeste is beginning to feel overwhelmed. She looks to other nursing colleagues for support. No one is available to help her manage the additional workload.

One day, while Dr. Schwartz is on vacation, he asks Celeste to see his wife's relative for a routine consultation. The patient's diabetes has been uncontrolled, and Dr. Schwartz believes she may benefit from using an insulin pump. Insulin pumps are one of Celeste's areas of expertise. She has become quite competent in educating patients on their proper use.

Throughout the visit with Dr. Schwartz's patient, Celeste is paged multiple times by the nursing staff and the emergency department with questions and requests for consults. She is distracted from her NP role yet manages to make it through the visit and arranges for a follow-up appointment with the client the next week. The client, however, appears annoyed with the constant interruptions.

Upon arriving at work the next morning, Celeste is informed that her patient had been admitted to the hospital through the emergency department the night before. Celeste panics, as she cannot recollect whether she instructed the client on the strategies needed to prevent potential complications related to the insulin pump. In fact, Celeste realizes she failed to give her any of the reference information that goes along with the equipment (which is still sitting on her desk) because she was so distracted.

Think about Celeste's decisions as you answer these yes/ no questions:

1. Is there a conflict in the institutional hierarchy at Celeste's workplace?
2. Should Celeste have informed Dr. Schwartz of her additional responsibilities?
3. Did Celeste's decision to assume the additional responsibilities adversely affect the care that she provided?
4. Did Celeste's decision put her client at risk?
5. Did Celeste put herself at risk?

Of course, the correct answer to each question is *yes*. There is certainly a conflict in the institutional hierarchy. Celeste should have informed Dr. Schwartz of the change in her workload. Her decision adversely affected the care she provided. Celeste has put her patient at risk for negative outcomes. She also could have put herself at risk for malpractice, and could have jeopardized both her job and her license.

Did this clinical scenario clarify why it is important that all parties understand to whom the NP ultimately reports? If Celeste had shared her concerns with Dr. Schwartz and Robert immediately, this incident might have been prevented. Further, it would have been best if Celeste's place in the organizational chart had been put in writing when she was hired.

=====*FAST FACTS in a NUTSHELL*

When the NP or others are uncertain as to whom the NP reports, problems may and likely will develop.

INDEPENDENT PRACTICE

One additional administrative issue needs to be briefly mentioned: starting an independent NP practice. I do not consider myself an expert in this area, as my NP career has not taken me down this path. If this is a journey you are considering, review some of the excellent resources on this aspect of NP practice.

My position is that a new NP is not prepared for independent practice right out of graduate school. No matter how seasoned a nurse or exceptional a student you are, some period of transition is necessary to attain competency in this new role. How much experience, you may ask? This is not an easy question to answer, but somewhere between 1 and 5 years—maybe more. The time required depends on the characteristics of the individual. Still, I fully respect and support NPs in independent practice. I wholeheartedly believe that NPs can and should run successful practices. I just do not think that the audience for this book is likely ready for this level of practice.

The novice NP may not be prepared for an independent practice site, as this role is best suited for the seasoned practitioner.

16

Discrimination

Discrimination can happen anywhere. Nurses and other health care professionals can be faced with discrimination that can interfere with providing appropriate care. Nurse practitioners (NPs) must understand the measures they can take to prevent being discriminated against and to ensure they are not discriminating against others.

This chapter clarifies types of discrimination NPs may face on the job. Ways to be protected from workplace discrimination are also presented. A case scenario is incorporated to clarify the risks associated with workplace discrimination.

In this chapter, you will learn:

1. How workplace discrimination may affect the NP
2. Ways of preventing workplace discrimination

WORKPLACE DISCRIMINATION AND THE NURSE PRACTITIONER

Many types of discrimination exist. Discrimination can be based on age, race, or gender, as well as a variety of other factors. One of the best ways to be protected from discrimination in the workplace is to join a union. A primary purpose of a union is to ensure that its members are treated fairly on the job. Unionized employees are also provided with a formal means of complaint if they feel they are being treated unfairly.

Are most NP job opportunities unionized? Some are, but many are not. Therefore, it is the responsibility of every NP to protect himself or herself against workplace discrimination.

Before accepting an NP position, be certain that the work environment does not support discriminatory practices. Review a new or potential employer's policy against discrimination on the job. Does a policy exist? If not, this is something to consider when accepting a new position. If the job is too good to pass up, accept it and then volunteer to create and lead a task force to create an institutional policy against workplace discrimination.

Again, return to the process of self-reflection. Have you ever felt discriminated against as a nurse? What factors were involved? The history of nursing as a female-dominated profession and medicine as a male-dominated profession make it likely that you may have felt some level of discrimination as a nurse.

═══════════════════════*FAST FACTS in a NUTSHELL*

NPs can play a key role in leading a task force to create policies to protect themselves from workplace discrimination.

AVOIDING OR ELIMINATING WORKPLACE DISCRIMINATION

The elimination of workplace discrimination is an evolutionary process. Increasing numbers of men are entering the nursing profession, and women are starting to outnumber their male colleagues in medical schools. I hope to see the day when men and women enter the medical and nursing professions equally because of a true understanding and passion for their respective fields—not because of traditional gender roles and stereotypes.

Consider the following scenario and answer the question at the end to see what you have learned in this chapter.

Will has been a successful oncology nurse for almost 20 years. He has just become a certified NP and accepted a position at a home health care agency. He is adjusting well to his new role and is getting acquainted with members of the experienced multidisciplinary team, many of whom have worked together for years.

Will's role does not require him to come to the agency daily, but he does so from time to time for team meetings and in-services. One day, as he is about to enter the conference room, he hears a group of female nurses laughing and encouraging one of their members to approach Will about dating her. Will's immediate supervisor, Grace, the patient care manager, is in the room during the discussion. Grace is not part of the conversation, but she does not address those participating. How should Will address this situation? (As you think about the question, consider what your answer would be if Will was female and the coworkers were male.)

1. Quit.
2. Ignore it.
3. Confront the participants.
4. Report his colleagues to their manager.
5. Make an official complaint through human resources.

The "correct" answer is option 5, depending on institutional policy.

Only Will can decide what course of action is right for him. He is an effective nurse and an asset to his new colleagues, who no doubt would not want him to quit. Ignoring the situation may work, but he may be faced with similar circumstances in the future. Confronting his coworkers may create an uncomfortable work environment. His manager is already aware of their behavior, as she was present. Her decision not to intervene may affect how she would handle the situation if Will came to her. As you can see, Will is faced with a complex problem. This situation could, in fact, be different if gender roles were reversed. This should not be so.

Everyone knows that coworkers often date. An adult's decision to date someone from the workplace is his or her own business, as long as it does not violate institutional policy. But remember your new role. It is possible, or even probable, that you may now be in a supervisory role over other nursing professionals. You need to be aware of the institutional policy to ensure you are not discriminated against and that you do not discriminate against others. This scenario demonstrates how the NP can become involved in a situation where workplace discrimination occurs.

===*FAST FACTS in a NUTSHELL*

- Circumstances exist in which discrimination can affect the NP in the workplace.
- The elimination of workplace discrimination is an evolutionary process.

17

Institutional Violence

Health care professionals, as well as those in other fields, are at a higher risk for violence at work. As professionals, nurse practitioners (NPs) need to identify situations that may increase their risk for being victimized and employ strategies to protect themselves. They must also protect themselves from stressors that could affect their own abilities to cope with anger or frustration and, in turn, cause them to act violently against others.

This chapter identifies reasons why NPs may be at risk for institutional violence. Scenarios in which the NP sets the stage to protect himself or herself from a variety of threats, with supporting rationales, are provided.

In this chapter, you will learn:

1. Pitfalls for institutional violence in health care
2. Why NPs may be at higher risk than other health care professionals

PROTECTING YOURSELF

Nurses are at risk for violence at work. Workplace violence may occur as a result of interactions with a coworker or when caring for a patient. Nurses and other health care professionals are also often faced with high levels of stress. This fact is well known and can result in burnout, addiction, and other behaviors that may, in turn, increase the risk for behaving violently.

Other important threats may increase the risk for work-related violence. Some of these include being alone with risky patients or visitors, terrorism, working during off hours, low staffing levels at certain times of day, and the availability of and access to certain medications. Effective strategies include recognizing or predicting dangerous situations and acting quickly and correctly if they occur. Institutions must put effective policies in place for their employees and train them to be aware of how to protect themselves and their colleagues.

===== FAST FACTS in a NUTSHELL

- Nurses and other health care professionals are often faced with high levels of stress.
- NPs must be aware of the risks of institutional violence and employ strategies to prevent them.

NURSE PRACTITIONER LEADERSHIP

As nursing leaders, NPs must play an active role in the prevention of threats that may adversely affect their practice. Violence is one of them. **If a policy does not exist in your place of employment or you do not believe the policy to be adequate, then take a stand.** Get involved. Help to create policies or modify existing ones. Start a committee. An excellent resource, and a good place to start, is the Occupational Safety and Health Administration (OSHA) *Guidelines for Preventing Workplace Violence for Health Care and Social Service Workers* (U.S. Department of Labor, OSHA, n.d.). Its overall recommendation is the creation and dissemination of a clear policy of zero tolerance for workplace violence.

Nurses are health care professionals who are well aware of their increased risk for violence at work. You learned about this in nursing school and perhaps through work-related programs and policies. The risk can vary depending on the setting and population with which one works.

===*FAST FACTS in a NUTSHELL*

NPs must play a leadership role in creating policies and developing programs to prevent institutional violence.

SITUATIONS OF INCREASED RISK

Two situations can possibly increase the risk of violence. The first occurs as NPs assume the role of independently managing patients in many practice settings. Thus, NPs are often alone with patients in an examination room. Common sense would dictate that there are times when this is not a good idea. Should an NP make a point never to go into an exam room alone with a patient? No. This is not practical and likely not possible in most busy practices or institutions.

However, NPs should be careful and use their best judgment. When in doubt, ask another staff member to accompany you. Do not evaluate a client alone in an examination room with a closed door if there is a known history of or suspected violence or the client is presently under the influence of drugs or alcohol. As you are well aware, there are some cases where clients with a psychiatric history may pose an increased risk as well. Keep this in mind and protect yourself.

You should also consider this risk when evaluating an unclothed member of the opposite sex. What am I talking about? Nurses take care of naked patients all the time, you are probably thinking. Yes, but in a different role. On a hospital floor or in the emergency department, you examine patients behind a curtain. Being alone behind a closed door is different. You need to be safe. Just keep these guidelines in mind in accordance with institutional policy.

Situations in which the NP is alone with a high-risk patient should be avoided.

Another scenario in which NPs are being placed at an increased risk for violence occurs when refusing to prescribe certain medications or complete specific forms (e.g., work excuses or disability paperwork). This is one of the only times when I (secretly) appreciate some of the restrictions placed on NPs. Some states restrict NPs' scope of prescriptive authority (particularly with controlled substances) and their ability to sign certain official paperwork. Each NP is responsible for becoming familiar with the policies in his or her state.

From experience, I know that some individuals may become argumentative or possibly violent if you refuse to prescribe certain medications or fill out a form in a particular way. Always tell a client that it is your obligation to comply with the law and the standards for practice. Do not comply with inappropriate requests. Use the "broken record" technique, as my mother always calls it. Do not argue. Just keep stating, clearly and professionally, that complying with the patient's request is breaking the law, and you will not break the law. Then politely excuse yourself from the situation.

My policy is that if the medication is warranted and is within my scope of practice, I will prescribe it, but I determine the dose, instructions, and the quantity. Clients, particularly those with some addictive behaviors, may try to manipulate you during questioning. Stick to the rules and your instincts. Your nursing background has taught you the red flags associated with particular types of patients. You can always check with the pharmacy to verify a client's medication history.

Be prepared for patients who present on weekends at urgent care settings—which often employ NPs—for a chronic health condition. This is a time when patients are unable to seek medical attention from their usual providers.

What should you do if they require a medication that has addictive properties? Clearly, the NP should not refuse to treat a patient who is in pain, anxious, or suffering from insomnia. However, one suggestion is to prescribe very small quantities of the addictive substance until the patient can follow up with his or her regular provider. Explain that this is in the patient's best interest and clearly document so in the chart. This way, the NP adheres to professional standards in providing care, but also complies with legal and ethical guidelines.

Another risk for violence occurs when an NP refuses to accede to a patient's request to be excused from work. Again, the level of risk is highly dependent on the setting, but NPs should be aware that employers are becoming increasingly more specific about their policies for excused work absences. For the most part, if a patient is sick enough to come in for a consultation, then some type of documentation of the visit is justifiable. If, in addition, the patient requests documentation excusing an additional day or two, NPs must use their judgment based on their evaluation and the patient's treatment course. In my practice, we use either computerized or carbon-copy work/school excuses, so documentation is always maintained in the client record.

Be aware, and be prepared. I have had countless encounters with clients who have been argumentative because they did not receive paperwork that suited their purposes. The same technique is recommended here. You decide. You follow the rules. Document appropriately and protect yourself. Whenever possible, an argumentative, or possibly even violent, patient should not be permitted back into the facility. Be certain a policy for such situations is in place. If it is not, work toward creating one.

As you read the following scenario, think about which of the two NPs, Barbara or Ross, followed the guidelines presented in this chapter pertaining to work-related violence.

Mr. G is a 30-year-old client with a known history of mental illness, substance abuse, and a chronic pain condition. He presents to the urgent health care center on a Sunday afternoon. His chief complaint is "back pain." He tells the nurse he needs refills of his medications (and provides her with a handwritten list). He also states that he needs some paperwork completed, as he has been out of work all week because of the pain. He was not able to get an appointment with his usual practitioner or his psychiatrist and needs to return to work in the morning as he has used up all of his sick time.

Barbara, an adult nurse practitioner (ANP) at the facility for 1 year, discusses the case with the nurse after reviewing the chart. She enters the examination room and closes the door, obtains a problem-focused history, and performs the related physical examination. She then explains to the client that she would need to consult with his psychiatrist and his primary care provider before refilling his medications and that she would be happy to provide him with an excused absence for the following morning to allow him time to seek the care that he needs. Barbara also agrees to refill a small quantity of one of his pain medications, once the dose is confirmed with his usual pharmacy, to ensure his comfort overnight.

Mr. G immediately begins to use profanity and becomes aggressive, kicking over the garbage can. He threatens to report the NP for refusing him care. He lunges at her, but stops himself, and then punches the wall. He turns and leaves the facility through an emergency exit door.

Now consider the same scenario and the approach taken by another practitioner. Ross has been a family nurse practitioner (FNP) at this same facility for 15 years. He has had multiple weekend encounters with Mr. G. Although Mr. G has never behaved violently, Ross understands that he possesses several known characteristics for violent behavior. He chooses to evaluate Mr. G in the examination room closest to the nurses' station and leaves the door slightly open. He asks a nurse to remain close by. Before evaluating Mr. G, he contacts the client's pharmacist as indicated on the client record and determines the correct names and doses of all of his medications, as well as the quantity and date they were last filled. Upon entering the room, Ross begins by stating: "Good to see you again Mr. G. I heard you were in pain, so

I did not want to keep you waiting and called your pharmacy to see what refills you needed. The pharmacist was kind enough to tell me that you just picked up all your medications last week, including your pain medications. So what was it that I could do for you today?" Mr. G shakes his head, mumbles something under his breath, and leaves.

Who do you feel best handled the patient?

The nursing code of ethics requires that NPs make every effort to help patients. Yet NPs must also protect themselves, their colleagues, and other patients. Although some elements of her approach were helpful and Barbara tried her best to help Mr. G, she may have put herself and others at risk. Ross gathered the information he needed and trusted his instincts that Mr. G would leave once he found out he would not be prescribed pain medication. Ross' approach was the more effective one.

FAST FACTS in a NUTSHELL

Stick to the rules and trust your instincts. Your nursing background has taught you the red flags for patient types that require special care in terms of possible violence.

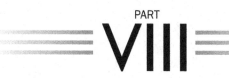

PART

VIII

Understanding Legal Issues

18

Contracts

The first legal issue a new nurse practitioner (NP) will face is the details of an employment contract. You should consider addressing the following items in a contract: salary and other benefits; practice hours and settings; malpractice insurance; tuition and other forms of reimbursement; policies for annual increases and reviews; and rules for termination of employment, including restrictive clauses. After completing this chapter, you should thoroughly understand the importance of this legal document; subsequent chapters then further explain the importance of each item.

In this chapter, you will learn:

1. What needs to be in your employment contract
2. Details on why these items are so important

THE DETAILS

The details of an employment contract are essential. In some cases, it might be prudent to have an attorney review the

TABLE 18.1 Recommended Items—Employment Contract

Salary (annual, hourly, performance-based, profit-sharing, overtime)

Benefits (health; vacation, holiday, sick, and personal time and coverage; pension)

Hours (office, hospital rounds, home care, nights, weekends, holidays, call)

Malpractice insurance, licensure

Tuition reimbursement, continuing education, journal subscriptions

Annual increases, reviews, rules for termination of employment

contract, but this is not usually necessary. A good place to start is to ask if you can review your mentor's contract. This may help you identify what is important for you and what might not be as important. Table 18.1 lists items that you should consider addressing in an employment contract. This list is, of course, not inclusive.

SALARY AND OTHER BENEFITS

Although there are many reasons why a registered nurse (RN) considers becoming an NP, a higher salary scale is probably one of the major motivations. A number of sources publish NP salary surveys, including *ADVANCE for Nurse Practitioners,* which reported the results of a questionnaire administered to collect data for its national salary survey from 2,889 NPs in 2013. Table 18.2 presents the average national NP salary for the years 1997 to 2013. Table 18.3 contrasts salaries (as of 2008) according to level of nursing education; however, a more recent 2011 survey revealed a much higher annual salary ($8,576) for doctorally prepared NPs. Table 18.4 compares salaries for NPs to those for other professionals. Table 18.5 contrasts NP salaries by practice setting, and Table 18.6 is a comparison by gender.

In addition to salary, benefits must be clearly delineated in your employment contract. Some of these may not

TABLE 18.2 Average National Nurse Practitioner Salary	
2013	$98,817
2012	$93,032
2011	$90,583
2010	$90,770
2009	$89,579
2008	$83,000
2007	$81,397
2005	$74,812
2003	$69,203
2001	$63,172
1999	$58,391
1997	$52,532

Source: Advance Healthcare Network (2013).

TABLE 18.3 Salary by Level of Nursing Education, 2008	
Doctoral degree	$84,786
Master's degree	$81,517

Source: Advance Healthcare Network (2013).

TABLE 18.4 Comparison to Other Professionals	
Physician assistant	$107,268
Nurse practitioner	$98,817

Source: Advance Healthcare Network (2013).

be negotiable, depending on institutional policies. Ask to review the employee handbook. Many benefits are standardized among all employees, particularly in large institutions, and certainly if the position will be overseen by a union.

TABLE 18.5 Nurse Practitioner Salary by Practice Setting, 2012

Academia	$88,211
Cardiology clinic	$88,900
Emergency department	$106,591
Endocrinology clinic	$89,974
Hospital	$96,523
Mental health	$101,444
Private practice	
Family	$90,600
Urgent care	$96,058
Women's health	$84,704
College health (12 month)	$82,832
Retail clinic	$88,027
Surgical setting	$96,923

Source: Advance Healthcare Network (2013).

TABLE 18.6 Salary by Gender

Male (8%)	$107,065
Female (92%)	$97,797

Source: Advance Healthcare Network (2013).

The most critical benefits to be included in an employment contract are health insurance and related benefits; vacation, holiday, personal, and sick time and coverage; pension opportunities; and or disability arrangements. In these economic times, you need to know all the terms of employment. How many paid days off are you permitted annually? What if you get sick? Many employers offer paid vacation and sick leave, yet leave it up to the employee to obtain his or her own replacement. Will this be feasible or practical? If you are scheduled to work on Thanksgiving Day and get sick, who will cover for you?

Pension or other types of retirement plans should be clear in an employment contract. Does the employer offer retirement plans? If so, what type(s)? Are the savings matched? Today, the media and other sources have empowered us to recognize the importance of planning for retirement. When I first joined the workforce, as is likely certain with many young employees, this was the last thing on my mind. This attitude needs to change.

===*FAST FACTS in a NUTSHELL*

- Besides salary, benefits must be clearly delineated in your employment contract.
- The most critical benefits to be included in an employment contract are health insurance and related benefits; vacation, holiday, personal, and sick time and coverage; pension opportunities; and disability arrangements.

HOURS ON THE JOB

This next topic can really affect your quality of life: the hours you will be expected to be at work. Where will you be expected to put in hours? In the office? In the hospital on rounds? What about home care? Probably even more important—when? Will you be required to work evenings? Nights? Weekends? Holidays? Participate in on-call schedules? How will this be compensated?

Your contract should specifically state the amount of any combination of these hours you will be required to work. For example, if the contract says "some weekend hours are mandated," what exactly does this mean? As low person on the totem pole, will you be expected to work every weekend? A contract that says "all employees are expected to work two

8-hour weekend shifts per month" is much clearer. Here, you will know the expectations right from the start.

Finally, what about overtime? Will you be a salaried or an hourly employee? Most professionals earn a salary. However, if your scheduled day is supposed to end at 8 p.m. and, week after week, you do not leave until 10 p.m. because of the demands of your new role, this could greatly affect your quality of life, as well as your bottom line. Sometimes, hourly payments could be a favorable scenario for you. At other times, they may not. Just be sure that you are clear on the terms and can live with them.

=== *FAST FACTS in a NUTSHELL*

When and where you will be expected to work should be written out in an employment contract and acceptable to both parties.

WHAT ELSE?

Malpractice insurance is another area to negotiate into an employment contract. Chapter 19 focuses on the importance of and various types of coverage offered. Here, however, just note that you can and should get your employer to cover your malpractice insurance. If this is a term that you and the employer agree on, get it in writing. How much will be covered? For how often? If this is important to you, it needs to be specific.

Tuition reimbursement and support for continuing education, conferences and related travel, and journal subscriptions are additional points to be negotiated in a thorough employment contract. It is not enough for an employer to tell you that these important activities will be covered. What is allowed, with the specific dollar amounts per year, should be put in writing. This may be standard from employee to employee, but it also may be negotiable.

Other elements to consider are the means and amounts of annual salary increases, and times and components of the review process. The review process may be standardized. It may be based on merit. Just be sure it is clear and acceptable to you. If it is not described in your contract, you will not have a leg to stand on if, as the years go by, your employer is not able or willing to renegotiate your salary. Times are tough, economically, and many institutions and practices are struggling. You need to protect yourself.

Finally, **the contract should specify very clearly the rules for termination of employment,** including restrictive clauses. As in any job, employers may not like you, and you may not like them. So, what happens if either party decides to move on?

Make sure you understand the ins and outs of the phraseology here, especially if you are interested in seeking employment at other institutions or practices that are seen as "the competition." For instance, if you are considering a new position, your contract may specify that you are not permitted to work within a specific geographical perimeter for a particular period of time. This is a common clause in employment contracts and may severely limit future career opportunities. I am not saying you must avoid it entirely—you may not be able to! Just be certain you are aware of the rules and agreeable to the terms.

If you need further proof of the importance of an employment contract, read this personal communication from a colleague:

> Practitioners should use caution in selecting a collaborating physician. I worked with one who was an excellent clinician and a great collaborator but never financially rewarded my positive contributions to the practice. I initially joined the practice at a low hourly rate because I was a new graduate. It then took years for me to negotiate a minimal salary increase, as no formal means of review or periodic increases were laid out in my employment contract. I advise all NPs to do their homework and research the current rate in their specialty area and geographical region. Bring in the hard copies of these documents as this may be beneficial. The handling

of licensure fees, malpractice insurance, supplies, and continuing education should also be clarified and put in writing.

=================================*FAST FACTS in a NUTSHELL*

Malpractice insurance and other forms of reimbursement, means of regular performance reviews and increases, and clarification of the terms for terminating employment, are essential elements of a well-written employment contract.

19

Malpractice

Years ago, in most malpractice cases, the plaintiff's attorney went after the physician for damages. At that time, physicians had the power, and they had the money. Today, everyone involved in care usually is named in the lawsuit. Nurse practitioners (NPs) are practicing at a completely different level than nurses. They are in charge, and they are making the decisions. It is possible or even likely that the physician has not even seen the patient in many cases. The NP may have been the primary provider managing the care of a client who has initiated a lawsuit.

This chapter explores the debate over maintaining your own personal protection liability insurance policy when you are already covered by policies provided by an employer or institution. Strategies for selecting a policy are reviewed.

In this chapter, you will learn:

1. Reasons to purchase personal liability insurance
2. What to look for in a policy

PERSONAL PROTECTION LIABILITY INSURANCE

Let me start by saying I have a personal protection liability insurance policy and have always maintained one. I think it is important. So do most practicing NPs and knowledge-able attorneys. There is, however, a debate over whether you should maintain your own policy when you are already covered by policies provided by an employer or institution. Either way, you need to be certain that you are aware of the risks and benefits of your decision.

The cost of the policy varies based on the company, your length of time in practice, coverage amount, specialty area, practice site(s), previous work history, and usual number of hours worked weekly. Currently, the expected cost can vary from several hundred to thousands of dollars per year. This is why this topic is so important and controversial.

Start by reviewing the policy offered by the company that currently insures you as a nurse. Then compare it with the competition. To help you begin, some companies to explore are presented in Table 19.1. This list is not, by any means, inclusive. There are many companies out there. It is your turn to do the research! Smaller, independent insurance companies or brokers may offer a policy that better meets your individual needs.

=FAST FACTS in a NUTSHELL

- The cost of the a policy will vary based on several factors, such as your length of time in practice, coverage amount, specialty area, practice site(s), previous work history, and usual number of hours to be worked weekly.
- Start by reviewing the policy offered by the company that currently insures you as a nurse.

HOW TO CHOOSE?

As always, talk to your preceptors, mentors, and colleagues in the field. Shop around—there is great variation in the

TABLE 19.1 Insurance Companies to Explore for Personal Liability Insurance

Nurses Service Organization (www.nso.com)

Proliability (www.proliability.com)

CM&F Group, Inc. (www.cmfgroup.com/insurance_products/ professional_liability_individual/nurse_practitioner.html)

level of coverage and pricing offered. See what you learned from this chapter by identifying which of the following statements is true or false.

1. The NP does not have to worry about being sued, as the physician is ultimately responsible for the patient.
2. It is not worthwhile to purchase personal protection liability (malpractice) insurance, as the hospital will always cover me.
3. The NP does not need to shop around, as all policies are similar and cost about the same.

Based on the key concepts presented in this chapter, the response to each statement is clearly *false.*

If you follow the strategies presented in this book, you may never be named in a lawsuit. Yet the statistics say otherwise. Increasing numbers of health care professionals are involved in lawsuits annually. You need to be realistic, and you need to protect yourself, your license, and your livelihood. Carry your own policy and negotiate that your employer pays for it.

=== *FAST FACTS in a NUTSHELL*

- Shop around! There is great variation in the level of coverage and pricing offered.
- Increasing numbers of health care professionals are involved in lawsuits annually.
- Carry your own policy and negotiate that your employer pays for it.

20

Avoiding Lawsuits

> *This chapter presents key strategies for protecting patients from injury or harm and, therefore, protecting nurse practitioners (NPs) from being sued—a critical aspect of the NP role. Most important are a clinician's strict adherence to standards of practice, diligent documentation, and adequate client follow-up.*

In this chapter, you will learn:

1. Recommended behaviors to avoid being sued
2. Principles of documentation for NPs

HELPING OTHERS AND PROTECTING PATIENTS FROM HARM

We go into nursing because of a desire to help others, which then becomes a professional path. Without this drive, or "calling," we would not survive our rough workdays and probably would not continue our nursing education.

Still, our work does put us in jeopardy of being sued. Our livelihoods and nursing careers are always at risk. Even after a lifetime of smart decisions that provide clients with excellent nursing care, the NP can be, and often is, sued.

WORK BEHAVIORS TO LIVE BY

You probably already know most of the basic actions discussed in this chapter. Taking a thorough patient history, performing a comprehensive physical exam, determining the appropriate course of action, and documenting your actions accordingly are nursing skills most readers have already mastered. What you do not know yet is how to apply these basic nursing behaviors at the advanced level required as an NP. Nurse practitioners do not solely report findings to the physician. They manage the care of their clients. As an NP, your decisions, and how you make them, are important: to you, your practice, and your client. This responsibility puts you at an increased risk for being sued.

What can you do to protect your patients and, therefore, yourself? I call my recommendations the "protect my patient . . . protect myself" protocol. Follow these simple guidelines with every patient you encounter.

Step one takes place during your history taking. I was once told by an NP faculty member that 80% of your diagnosis comes from the patient history you take, 15% from the physical examination, and 5% from diagnostic testing. At the time, I did not believe it. What did she mean? How could only 15% come from the physical component, which then seemed like the most critical part of the NP–patient interaction?

As a seasoned practitioner, I now completely agree. The quantity and quality of the questions you ask will guide your physical exam. They will also direct you to some possible differential diagnoses, tests you may consider ordering, and the overall treatment plan for effective management.

The following example illustrates step one of my "protect my patient . . . protect myself" protocol. The client, a 40-year-old woman, presents with chest pain. Some key things you would initially want to know are the duration of symptoms and the location of the pain, including its intensity; whether it radiates and, if so, to where; if is it constant or intermittent; what causes it, what alleviates it; and what accompanies it (e.g., shortness of breath, nausea, vomiting, diaphoresis, dizziness, cough, heartburn). You should also ask the client to describe the pain (i.e., sharp, dull, burning, stabbing). If the symptoms have come and gone for 2 years, your approach would be different than if she reports sudden onset a few hours ago.

Next, you would want to know her family history. If her mother died at age 37 of "unknown causes," then your approach might change quickly. Of course, you would also want to know the client's own medical, surgical, and social history. For instance, if she had a complete hysterectomy 10 years ago and has lost some of the cardioprotective benefits of estrogen, this is an important consideration. If she has hypertension, diabetes, or hyperlipidemia, you would also approach the case slightly differently. Has she experienced any recent trauma? Begun new activities or exercise? This list is not inclusive, but it is a start.

The client's answers to these questions would guide further probing. For example, if she then complains of heartburn, you would evaluate for other gastrointestinal signs and symptoms. If she complains of an accompanying cough, you would seek more information about other respiratory signs and symptoms.

Most of this you already know from your nursing background. But now, you need to put it all together in a slightly different way than you did as a nurse.

Your documentation is also taken to an advanced level. Thus, **step two** of "protect my patient . . . protect myself" is **to chart.** If you are using a SOAP note (subjective, objective, assessment, plan), this data all goes under subjective information (S). It is important that you document the negatives

here, as well. For instance, "Denies: nausea, vomiting, shortness of breath, diaphoresis, radiation," and so on. Here, you
must include the most serious negatives that are related to
the chief complaint. In this case, it would be the cardiac
findings, of course. If the client ends up with costochondri-
tis or reflux, this is obviously not as serious as if she is having an acute myocardial infarction (MI). Documentation is
how you protect yourself. If you ask but do not write the
client's answer down, it is not considered done.

Have you noticed anything striking about the preceding
description? You have not yet touched the client: All of this
information has been gathered during the history taking!

=== *FAST FACTS in a NUTSHELL*

- The quantity and quality of the questions you ask
  while taking a history will guide you in the overall
  treatment plan for effective management.
- Always document the patient's history.

Now you are ready to assess the client, or gather objective
data (the O of the SOAP note). **Your thorough history guides
the parameters for step three—the physical assessment.**
Obviously, assessing this client for abnormal or irregular
heart sounds is critical. However, cardiac sounds can be normal in someone having an MI. Breath sounds and abdominal
and musculoskeletal assessment are also important in this
particular clinical case.

Be thorough in your exam. Consider all possibilities. For
example, as you are completing your examination of this
female client, she describes a blistery rash that appeared on
the left side of her chest a few days ago. Although dermato-
logic conditions were likely not included in your initial differential diagnoses, if you did not now lift up her shirt you might
miss the grouped vesicular lesions (probably shingles) on her
chest. You may have heard it said that the phrase "within
normal limits" (WNL) can also mean "we never looked," so
ensure that your problem-focused exam is comprehensive.

Step four is recording your pertinent assessment findings. Obviously, you will document abnormal assessment findings, but you should not simply write "normal" for everything else. Think of the differentials going through your mind, and also document the negatives from your exam. For instance, if the pain is not elicited with palpation of the chest wall or with movement, document this. If no discomfort is reported upon palpation of the epigastric region, record this too. If the lungs are free from adventitious sounds, this requires documentation. This is an example of how careful, conscientious charting protects your patient. It also protects you from being sued.

═══════════════════════════════════*FAST FACTS in a NUTSHELL*

- Conduct a careful and complete physical assessment.
- Be certain to document abnormal, as well as normal, findings that are relevant to your differential diagnoses.

Step five of the "protect my patient . . . protect myself" protocol **occurs during the assessment and planning phases (A and P).** Your diagnoses will guide your treatment plan. Every diagnosis in your plan needs to have a corresponding action. For example, if you are considering a cardiac etiology, your next step may be an ECG. (Even if I was leaning toward the pain being noncardiac in nature, I would want to include a normal ECG on the chart before proceeding). If you are concerned about respiratory symptoms, a chest x-ray may become part of the workup. A number of other diagnostics, such as blood or a breath test, may also become part of the workup for this patient. Remember to be certain that each part of your workup matches your diagnoses.

The proper use of pharmacotherapy, diagnostics, and referrals is addressed in Chapters 25 through 27, but these components are mentioned here because, if improperly handled, they can become the basis of a lawsuit. Ordering the correct medication, appropriate diagnostic test, and possibly an important consultation with a specialty provider or a referral to the emergency department protects you and your patient. Step six is, again, proper documentation.

============================*FAST FACTS in a NUTSHELL*

- Your diagnoses will guide your treatment plan.
- Again, document your assessment and your handling of pharmacotherapy, diagnostics, and referrals.

Step seven is one of the most important actions—what you told or taught the patient before he or she left. This should not be difficult to remember, as this is what nurses do best! Let's say the client denied any additional cardiac symptoms, had no past or family history, and a negative ECG. She had been gardening over the weekend, the pain appeared to be musculoskeletal in nature, and her examination was unremarkable, aside from pain on palpation of the chest wall. You would likely prescribe a nonsteroidal anti-inflammatory drug (NSAID), instruct her on symptomatic therapy, and ask her to follow up in a week if still symptomatic. This should all be documented accordingly.

My chart *always* includes that the client has been educated on the signs and symptoms that indicate the need to return to the office or seek urgent care, and that the client verbalizes understanding of these instructions. A general statement, such as "client instructed on and verbalized understanding of s/s to return to clinic or emergent s/s to seek urgent care," would suffice here. You might also add, "if chest pain changes or worsens in any way, client understands to seek emergency services." Again, what you write here depends on the history and physical assessment findings you have obtained. If anyone subsequently reviews the chart, it will be clear what you taught your patient.

============================*FAST FACTS in a NUTSHELL*

It is imperative that you document any education you provide to the client.

Step eight is optional, but highly recommended—a follow-up phone call. It is neither expected nor practical to make a follow-up call to every patient you see. It is possible to do so, however, for the one or two patients about whom you may be concerned.

My rule of thumb is as follows: If I think about a patient after I have left the office, as many of us do, then consider a follow-up phone call. We all wake up in the middle of the night thinking, "I should have rechecked that patient's blood pressure," or, "Did I ask him if he had any allergies?" If you are concerned, then trust your intuition. If the client's condition is worsening or not improving, you may need to change your treatment plan. Without following up, you might not know there has been a change.

Studies show that if a patient feels you are truly concerned, he or she is less likely to sue you. Of course, this is not the only reason to be conscientious, but it fits within the context of this chapter. Finally, if you choose to complete step eight, what will step nine be? Well, of course, to document it.

══════════════ *FAST FACTS in a NUTSHELL*

Trust your intuition and follow up accordingly.

DOCUMENT, DOCUMENT, DOCUMENT

Nurses are well aware of the critical nature of proper documentation. We learned this in Nursing 101. This point is reinforced at various places throughout this book. We can examine some comprehensive documentation strategies through the following example.

Pregnancy is generally a healthy state. In most cases, a pregnant women and her fetus will remain healthy. Yet, obstetricians are often sued for malpractice because of an increased risk for adverse outcomes. Even if you elect not to work in obstetrics, pregnant patients present to a variety of other settings for symptoms or conditions that may occur concurrently. Nurse practitioners need to be aware of concepts related to the management of a pregnant patient.

One example of a challenge facing NPs managing pregnant patients is prenatal screening. Today, a wide variety of prenatal tests are available to facilitate the proper care of a pregnant woman and her fetus. Some are required, but most are recommended. Most clients comply with the recommended prenatal screening tests. However, some do not. They may choose to forgo testing for financial, religious, or other reasons.

I recently asked a colleague, who is a woman's health NP, how she protects her clients and herself when presented with this issue. She cited thorough education and clear documentation as the key strategies. For example, she counsels her clients about the risk factors for certain chromosomal abnormalities, as well as the risks of the various recommended screening tests. She asks them to verbalize understanding of such risks. All of these actions are then carefully documented. If the client chooses to forgo the recommended procedure(s) and the child is born with an abnormality, the practitioner will be protected.

Overall, there are some basic things that patients expect and deserve from you. Patients are entitled to safe, effective practice. They expect their practitioner to be accurate. They expect you to be knowledgeable and skillful. They expect you to know your limits. They expect you to be accountable. If you follow these guidelines and provide your clients with the care they deserve within the NP scope of practice, then the likelihood of being sued will be greatly diminished.

=== FAST FACTS in a NUTSHELL

Proper documentation is one of the most important aspects in protecting yourself from being sued.

21

Dos and the Don'ts:
Electronic Health Records

This chapter presents strategies for effective electronic recordkeeping by nurse practitioners (NPs). Benefits of adopting electronic health records (EHR) are presented, as are potential risks of improper use. The relationship between quality of care and the proper use of EHR is further described for the reader.

In this chapter, you will learn:

1. What role EHR plays in the provision of quality advanced nursing care
2. Why NPs must adapt their documentation strategies for effective electronic recordkeeping

ELECTRONIC HEALTH RECORDS AND SUCCESS FOR NURSE PRACTITIONERS

Change is difficult and, at times, scary. However, throughout history, nurses have adapted to change. Electronic documentation is an important element of most nursing practice settings today. The EHR is here to stay. Your year of birth or previous exposure to and comfort level with technology may be the best predictors of your ability to adapt to these electronic record-keeping systems. Regardless, all nursing professionals must make themselves aware of the benefits and risks of using electronic documentation. Congruently, we must develop fluency in the proper use of the system we are expected to utilize to document care. **Essentially, it is the responsibility of the practicing NP to make the commitment to learning how to use electronic recordkeeping systems efficiently and effectively.**

EHR must be incorporated into the provision and management of high-quality advanced practice nursing care. The proper use of these systems may allow for easier access to the medical record, proficiency in receiving and reviewing diagnostic reports, enhanced communication between providers, prompt referral to specialty providers when necessary, and a wealth of other aspects of effectively coordinated health care services. EHR systems can play a key role in collecting, organizing, and interpreting data so that health care outcomes can be determined and reported.

EHR also permit the provider to visualize the patient record instantly so that important data such as problem lists, immunization history, and medications are at the clinicians' fingertips (Green, Wendland, Carver, Rinker, & Mun, 2012). Access to patient data from home or other practice sites is an additional feature that EHR systems offer to the provider. The use of EHR systems will be mandated; thus, the practicing nurse must maintain currency on these standards of today's practice environment, for example, through immersion in strategies to become proficient in proper use, and by keeping abreast of technological trends. EHR systems are just one example of how technological trends are evolving to address today's health care environments. **Technology is now a major force affecting most aspects of today's ever-changing, ever-challenged health care system.**

=== *FAST FACTS in a NUTSHELL*

EHR help to facilitate effective coordination of care and promote improved quality of health care outcomes.

The benefits of EHR are many. The elimination of errors due to illegible writing, decreased storage space required for charts, and improved ease of access—both on-site and remotely—are just some examples of the benefits of electronic recordkeeping. E-prescribing, advancements in billing and coding, and timely reimbursement are, perhaps, the greatest benefits. Drop-down menus, check lists, templates, and opportunities for narrative notation are some of the features these systems provide to facilitate user ease.

ISSUES IN EHR IMPLEMENTATION

Cost is a factor when adopting an electronic recordkeeping system. Up-front costs, as well as training time and system maintenance, must be factored into budgeting. There are also risks associated with improper use of these systems. First and foremost, as in handwritten documentation, if something is not documented it is not considered done. Further, I have found that the learning curve in gaining facility with documentation via EHR systems can vary greatly depending on the program and setting. Some programs can be simple to learn and use while others may be much more complex. The NP must actively participate in training to facilitate the transition to electronic documentation. Ample training time, both before and during initial use, and the availability of support and resources are key components for success.

=====FAST FACTS in a NUTSHELL

- EHR are here to stay.
- Nursing professionals must be certain to possess competency in all aspects of effective electronic documentation.

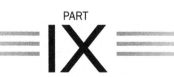

PART

IX

Collaboration

22

The Collaborative Agreement

Collaboration with a physician is an important part of nurse practitioner (NPs) practice. In most states, it is required. Having a physician available, whether in person, by phone, or online, is important particularly for those who are new to the NP role. This chapter defines and describes the collaborative agreement. It includes the required components of such a legal document, as well as some additional recommended items.

In this chapter, you will learn:

1. Why NPs need to collaborate
2. Essential components of the collaborative agreement

WHY COLLABORATE?

One of the single most important reasons the NP is required to have a collaborative agreement is to prescribe medications. In most settings, to practice in the role in accordance with the scope of practice, the NP must perform this important function. In a number of states, NPs have been granted the authority to practice without a collaborative agreement. This will be further discussed in Chapter 24.

The NP's ability to manage patients autonomously is based on the regulation that the NP works in collaboration with a physician, but the level of that collaboration is highly variable. There are some completely acceptable scenarios in which the NP and collaborating physician rarely see one another, and the collaborative agreement is, essentially, a formality.

For instance, an NP-directed practice will likely have a physician who has agreed to oversee the NPs in collaboration, although the physician does not directly participate in patient care. On the other hand, there are also practice settings where the NP and the MD work together side-by-side on a regular basis. The relationship depends on the work environment and the comfort level of both parties.

═══════════════════*FAST FACTS in a NUTSHELL*

- To prescribe in some states, the NP is required to have a collaborative agreement with a physician.
- The NP's level of collaboration with a physician varies greatly.

ESSENTIAL COMPONENTS OF COLLABORATION

The components of the collaborative agreement vary from state to state. Some agreements are quite specific, while others are rather general, but some items are always required. These begin with the names and proper titles of the parties involved and the locations of the sites where the NP will practice. The agreement must be signed (by both parties and a witness), dated, and renewed annually.

The agreement must also include the standards of care that the NP will be expected to follow, which are not the same in all collaborations. Specific diagnoses that the NP will manage should also be described. This is sometimes referred to as "cookie-cutter medicine," but I have not practiced with these types of guidelines. Usually, the collaborative agreement lists a number of general resources or references to which the NP can refer, such as a primary care manual. The NP is expected to practice in accordance with these guidelines.

Another critical part of this document is the facilities' regulations for prescribing. Again, this can be specific or quite broad. Here, computer-based resources or reference books can also be listed. The NP is required to manage patients and prescribe in accordance with these guidelines.

FAST FACTS in a NUTSHELL

- Components of the collaborative agreement vary from state to state.
- Some important components of the collaborative agreement include the names and titles of involved parties, date of renewal, practice site location, and guidelines for practice.

23

Selecting a Collaborating Physician

There are some guidelines that specify what to look for when selecting a collaborating physician, as this is a key individual in your practice. Ideally, your collaborating physician will have worked with nurse practitioners (NPs) before. This is particularly helpful in ensuring he or she is aware of the role, its abilities, and its limitations.

A physician who has already worked with NPs is well aware of the many benefits they bring to a practice. Other important attributes, such as the approachability of this key individual, are also presented. This is particularly important for the novice NP who may require more support in the transition to the new role.

In this chapter, you will learn:

1. Some characteristics to look for in a collaborating physician
2. Why selecting a collaborating physician is so important

WHAT TO LOOK FOR

Working with a collaborating physician who has worked with NPs before is the ideal. There is, however, no reason why you cannot and should not engage in a collaborative practice with a physician who is new to the experience. But, in this case, it may become your responsibility to educate him or her on the NP role.

The personality of this key individual, particularly for a novice NP, may be critical. Depending on your nursing background, experience, and comfort level in the new role, you may have a lot of questions. It is important to emphasize that you may be working very closely with this individual and need to work well together. I have known many NPs who joined a practice and left shortly after because the collaborating physician was not a good match for them.

Consider the following questions in making your decision by answering yes or no.

1. Do you view this individual as approachable?
2. In your opinion so far, does this individual understand the role of the NP?
3. Has this individual worked with NPs before?
4. Does he or she seem open to negotiation?
5. Did you feel comfortable during the hiring process?

If you answered no to more than two questions, consider exploring other employment options. The importance of a positive working relationship with this key individual cannot be overemphasized.

Chapter 22, on the collaborative agreement, mentioned a scenario in which the NP does not directly work alongside the collaborating physician. This may not be the best relationship for a new NP. **A novice needs support and direction.** At the same time, however, if other mentor(s) are directly available, such as experienced NPs, this sort of collaborative relationship could work out fine.

- A collaborating physician should be approachable and understand the role of the NP.
- A novice NP, who needs support and direction, may be more comfortable with a scenario in which he or she works directly alongside the collaborating physician.

AN IMPORTANT DECISION

Ideally, new NPs will work side-by-side with a collaborating physician. In doing so, they will learn the physician's practice style and begin to develop their own. As a novice NP, you will probably have many questions, and your collaborating physician will guide you in finding answers and identifying resources. You will become more independent in time.

I was fortunate to have an approachable, supportive collaborating physician during my first year as a practicing NP. He had had previous experience working with an NP, knew the role and scope of practice, and understood its limitations. He was patient and had a good sense of humor—always a plus!

═══════════*FAST FACTS in a NUTSHELL*

Ideally, novice NPs should work side-by-side with their collaborating physicians.

24

Collaborative Practice:
Harmonious or Burdensome?

This chapter focuses on key issues in the debate about the necessity of collaborative practice for nurse practitioners (NPs). Some rationales for collaboration are presented as well as reasons why this option is or is not favorable for the practicing NP. The current state of collaborative practice in the United States is discussed, and issues related to collaboration are explored.

In this chapter, you will learn:

1. What collaboration is and what it means for NPs
2. Why collaborative practice can be viewed as a harmonious relationship or a burdensome one

WHAT IS COLLABORATION?

Collaboration is an important process. According to the Centers for Medicare and Medicaid Services, collaboration is a process in which an NP works with one or more physicians to deliver health care services within the scope of the practitioner's expertise, with medical direction and appropriate supervision as provided for in jointly developed guidelines or other mechanisms as provided by the law of the state in which the services are performed (AMDA, n.d.).

IS COLLABORATION NECESSARY?

As previously discussed, collaborative practice can be an essential part of the transition into the NP role. Perhaps effective collaboration could be perceived as the most important factor. However, the regulation of this relationship has caused some controversy in recent times. For instance, many states do not require NPs to collaborate with a physician, and regulations on practice are quite variable from state to state. Greipel (2014) has reported that 19 states and the District of Columbia now allow NPs to practice independently in the United States, whereas another 19 states require a physician agreement for some aspects of management, such as prescribing controlled substances. This author goes on to report that increased efforts to remove restrictions on independent NP practice have faced opposition.

═══════════════════════════════*FAST FACTS in a NUTSHELL*

Nineteen states permit independent practice in the United States and another 19 require a physician agreement for practice.

The American Association of Nurse Practitioners (AANP, n.d.) defines the parameters of full practice, reduced practice, and restricted practice as follows:

Level of Practice	Definitions
Full	State practice and licensure law provides for NPs to evaluate patients, diagnose, order and interpret diagnostic tests, initiate and manage treatments—including prescribe medications—under the exclusive licensure authority of the state board of nursing. This is the model recommended by the Institute of Medicine and National Council of State Boards of Nursing.

Level of Practice	Definitions
Reduced	State practice and licensure law reduces the ability of nurse practitioners to engage in at least one element of NP practice. State requires a regulated collaborative agreement with an outside health discipline in order for the NP to provide patient care.
Restricted	State practice and licensure law restricts the ability of a nurse practitioner to engage in at least one element of NP practice. State requires supervision, delegation, or team management by an outside health discipline in order for the NP to provide patient care.

Source: AANP (n.d.).

The NP must be cognizant of the level of practice in his or her state and must practice accordingly.

The American Medical Association (AMA) has called for physician-led health care teams in place of autonomy for NPs, while the fact remains that the physician shortage prohibits adequate numbers of physicians from serving as collaborators (Greipel, 2014) and, further, the Institute of Medicine (IOM) has recommended that NPs be granted permission to practice to the full extent of their training. It is quite apparent that this debate will continue.

So how can you as you, as a recent NP, effectively contribute to the resolution of this issue? As previously discussed, for a newly practicing NP, a supportive collaborating physician may be one of the greatest factors in successful transition into the NP role. Stay informed and become active in your professional organizations.

TEST YOURSELF

Answer the following question to see what you have learned in this chapter. Which of the following NPs would *least* benefit from a collaborating physician?

1. Ashley, a new NP who graduated from a BSN-to-DNP program less than 6 months ago

2. Jackie, a seasoned NP who works in a state where a written collaborative agreement is mandatory for advanced nursing practice
3. William, a certified NP for 1 year, who recently left a nursing management position in an acute care setting for a fast-paced, inner city primary care clinic
4. Benjamin, an NP who has practiced in primary care for 5 years in a state that does not mandate collaboration, and who is also a recent DNP graduate

Correct answer: 4.
In evaluating the possible answers, consider the following:

1. A new NP would most benefit from a strong relationship with a collaborating physician.
2. If collaboration is mandatory, an NP *must* adhere to state regulations.
3. An NP in a new practice setting with less than 1 year of experience in the role would benefit from collaborative practice.
4. An experienced NP who is practicing in a state where collaboration is not a requirement for independent practice would least benefit from a formalized collaborative agreement. **Informal collaboration with a physician can benefit all practicing NPs.**

========================*FAST FACTS in a NUTSHELL*

Collaborative practice can be beneficial to some NP–physician dyads. It can, however, be burdensome in some states where collaboration is required and is not desirable to the NP.

PART

X

You're in Charge

25

Prescriptive Authority

One of the most important functions of a nurse practitioner (NP) is the ability to prescribe. This is an enormous responsibility. Prescribing is a different skill from solely administering medications. You will comprehend these differences after completing this chapter.

Being in charge is often intimidating, particularly to a new NP. In this chapter key resources needed to survive are shared. Evaluating your readiness to prescribe is presented as an essential component of NP practice. Ways to do so are described.

In this chapter, you will learn:

1. Guidelines for NP prescriptive practice
2. Ways to evaluate your readiness to prescribe
3. Useful resources for the new prescriber

MY REALITY

I can recall my very first day as a family nurse practitioner (FNP) working in a fast-paced, inner-city, primary/urgent care practice as if it were yesterday. Soon after my arrival, the office staff realized that no one had remembered to order my prescription pads. My collaborating physician "graciously" took out one of his pads. He proceeded to sign each and every one, handed the pad to me, and then pointed to an examination room to alert me that my first patient was waiting.

What, no orientation? No hand holding? No one was watching over me? How could this be? This was an eye-opening experience (at least for me). Some may refer to it as "baptism by fire."

Whatever you call it, it fast became my reality. I was now in charge. You, the NP, similarly are now the diagnostician and the prescriber. You have knowledge of pharmacology, but implementing an order is much different from writing one yourself.

No one will double check you (except maybe your local pharmacy computer system, if you are lucky). You are in charge. It sometimes is scary (okay, all the time for the first few months). Yes, you will have questions. Other, more experienced NPs, physicians, and pharmacists; the *Physician's Desk Reference* (*PDR*) and other drug books; downloadable references; apps and websites; and pharmaceutical company representatives (a.k.a. drug reps) will all be your allies as you assume this new role of the prescriber.

=== *FAST FACTS in a NUTSHELL*

- You, the NP, are now the diagnostician and the prescriber.
- Other NPs, MDs, pharmacists, pharmaceutical company representatives, books, and technology-based references will serve as important resources.

SO, ARE YOU READY?

Use the following quiz to test your knowledge about the NP's role as prescriber. Indicate whether each statement is true or false.

1. You do not have to worry when you prescribe as your collaborating physician is ultimately responsible and will double check you.
2. If you are too busy to confirm a medication dosage, you should not worry as the pharmacist has the ability to do so.
3. The number of refills you provide for the patient is not as important as the other elements of the prescription.
4. You do not need to worry about your handwriting. Have you seen some doctors' prescriptions?
5. It is important to spell the patient's name correctly and put the date on the prescription.
6. The correctly spelled medication name, dose, route, and frequency of administration, along with additional instructions when pertinent, must be provided.
7. The exact number or volume to be dispensed must also be included, as well the number of refills permitted.

Answers/Rationales:

1. *False:* It is you, the prescriber, who is ultimately responsible for all prescribing decisions. It is not likely that your collaborating physician or anyone else, for that matter, will double check you. Your decisions are critical.
2. *False:* Although the pharmacist should check dosages and may contact you for confirmation or clarification, it is the prescribers' responsibility to ensure that all of the essential components of a prescription are included.
3. *False:* The number of refills is a critical part of the prescription. Patients may ask for a refill on an antibiotic, for example, so they do not have to come back if the symptoms persist or reoccur. This is not a good idea. We all know why. If you ask your client to return in a few weeks to recheck blood pressure and then provide several refills of an antihypertensive, the client may not comply with your instruction.
4. *False:* Of course this is ridiculous. Many institutions and practices are getting away from the handwritten prescription and moving toward computer-printed prescriptions.

This is the best way to avoid errors related to poor handwriting. As nurses, we are all well aware of the risks of poor handwriting.

5. *True:* For the patient to fill the prescription, particularly using a prescription drug plan, his or her name must be spelled correctly. You will save the patient, and yourself, time and a headache if you comply with this. A prescription needs a date. Without one, you are allowing the patient to fill it at their discretion, not on your recommendation.

6. *True:* Each and every item described in this question is a critical element of a correctly written prescription.

7. *True:* You must write the quantity of the medication to be dispensed. It is also a safe feature to write out the number of refills. If the prescription is not permitted to be refilled, I recommend you write out the word "none." Never write a number "1," as this can easily be changed.

How did you do? If you responded incorrectly to any of these statements, review the guidelines to writing a prescription in a pharmacology textbook. Other useful references are provided in Table 25.1.

RESOURCES

Every prescriber should have up-to-date and detailed resources available. Medications change all the time. It is your responsibility to keep current and stay informed. The latest edition of the *PDR*, mentioned earlier, is the "gold standard" for prescribing. (I, of course, appeal to the publishers

---

TABLE 25.1 Nurse Practitioner Prescribing References

U.S. Nurse Practitioner Prescribing Law: A State-by-State Summary (www.medscape.com/viewarticle/440315)

Position Statement on Nurse Practitioner Prescriptive Privilege (www.aacn.org/WD/Practice/Docs/PositionStatementPrescriptive Authority.pdf)

---

to modify the title to the "Prescriber's Desk Reference," as it is not just physicians who utilize the resource.) Every practice needs to have a *PDR* and access to a variety of web-based resources reflecting the specialty area.

You should also use the *Nurse Practitioner's Prescribing Reference (NPPR)* (www.haymarket.com/monthly_prescribing_reference/multi/nppr_usa_magazine/default.aspx). Published quarterly, this manual is available at no charge to licensed NPs. It fits in your pocket and offers a quick way to check spelling, dosages, and dosing instructions. It is grouped by type of medication (e.g., diabetic agents or antiviral medications), so you can also use it to compare medications. It also includes charts, such as comparisons of products for nicotine addiction or bacterial coverage of antibiotics. Did I mention this is all free?

Another handy reference is the *Pocket Pharmacopeia*, which is available in several formats and is updated annually (www.tarascon.com/products/details.aspx/02670-2). It is part of a series of related pocket-sized references. This guide provides the user with critical aspects of and information for prescribing. It is not free, but it is affordable.

One additional beneficial resource is the *Sanford Guide to Antimicrobial Therapy* (www.sanfordguide.com/). This guide for prescribing antibiotics is updated annually and is very helpful in selecting the best agent for a specific pathogen or condition. Web-based versions are also now available.

Additional computerized prescribing resources are also available. However, it is important that the novice practitioner be extremely careful when using the web as a resource. The references described above were useful to me as a student and a new practitioner. Today there are a wealth of apps and web-based programs available. It is not within the scope of this book to critique them. Downloadable applications, such as *Epocrates,* which is free, provide the prescriber with the most up-to-date information that is essential for prescriptive practice (www.epocrates.com). A number of other programs, some free and some fee based, can also be downloaded. You need to familiarize yourself with these resources. Prescriber information is changing all the time.

It is up to you, the prescriber, to stay current and prescribe precisely and accurately according to practice standards.

FAST FACTS in a NUTSHELL

- Medications change all the time, so it is your responsibility to keep current and stay informed.
- Familiarize yourself with both print and computer-based resources.

26

Diagnostics

This chapter describes the proper role of diagnostic testing in facilitating the development of an effective nurse practitioner (NP). Clinical examples will be used for explanatory purposes, but this is not a clinical chapter. Rather, it will prepare you to understand the proper role of diagnostic testing in thoroughly evaluating the clients you serve.

It is not reasonable, practical, or cost efficient to order extensive, expensive diagnostic testing on every client. This chapter explores how to find the right balance between reasonable and necessary tests and how to protect your patients and yourself by ordering them.

In this chapter, you will learn:

1. The importance of referring your clients for diagnostic testing when indicated
2. Guidelines to determine the necessity of ordering a diagnostic test(s)

THE IMPORTANCE OF A DIAGNOSTIC TEST

The proper ordering of various types of diagnostic tests is a key element of effective client management. To help clarify this point, consider the following clinical case example, which was presented by one of my NP students. It was an eye-opening case for me, and I think it will be for you as well.

Mrs. Jones, age 48, was complaining of persistent headaches (longer than 2 weeks). She had no relevant past medical history, family history, or social history factors and took no medications. The pain was intermittent but severe at times in the frontal, temporal, and occipital regions. She reported being under a great deal of stress at work and at home, as she was caring for her elderly mother with Alzheimer's disease. She denied fever, illness, or other neurological symptoms. Physical examination was unremarkable.

Overall, the initial workup and plan of care for a headache varies. Depending on the comfort level of the practitioner, this may range from a variety of pharmacological and nonpharmacological interventions to some diagnostic testing. Because of the recent increase in stress in this client, the practitioner might have recommended stress reduction and medication management, clearly instructing the client to return for a thorough workup if symptoms worsened, changed, or persisted. At that time, the client would receive additional diagnostic testing, such as bloodwork or imaging studies. Later, a specialty consult might also be indicated (see Chapter 27). This is a cost-effective approach in line with the standards of care for a low-risk client with no past medical history and a normal physical examination.

In this case, the seasoned NP preceptor trusted her instincts and did a complete workup, including imaging studies. Within 24 hours, the patient was diagnosed with an aggressive brain tumor. This dramatic case exemplifies the necessity of diagnostic testing in certain circumstances. I take my hat off to this practitioner for her ability to sense a problem and intervene quickly.

Because this aspect of practice is so critical to the NP role, another clinical example is included to emphasize the decision-making process involved. This case was not as serious as the previous one, but it stresses the other side of diagnostic testing—when not to order tests!

Miss Brown was a 24-year-old elementary school teacher who presented to a walk-in, urgent care center with a 48-hour history of fever—maximum oral temperature of 102 degrees—and some minor fatigue. She denied any other symptoms (constitutional, respiratory, gastrointestinal, genitourinary, dermatological, neurological, etc.). She had no medical history of serious illness. Her physical examination was unremarkable other than a 101.7-degree temperature. She was pleasant, cooperative, and in no apparent distress. Her previous health, age, and likely occupational exposure led me to a diagnosis of a viral syndrome.

Because I always try to trust a patient's instincts, I believed there was a reason she had presented so concerned about her fever. I did some routine bloodwork, which included a complete blood count (CBC). When I returned early the next morning, her chart was waiting with other urgent results. Results were normal except that her white blood cell count was 22,000 cells per microliter. I was able to reach her right away and had her come right back into the office.

At this time, she was weaker and appeared to be slightly dehydrated (probably from the persistent high fevers). I probed further and her urinalysis was normal. Next I ordered a chest x-ray (CXR), which revealed a large left lower lobe infiltrate. Pneumonia was probably causing her fever, and I treated her with an appropriate antibiotic. She responded well and her overall outcome was excellent.

What could I have done to better manage this clinical case? Well, looking back on it now, I still believe—nothing!

I was relieved that I trusted my instincts and ordered the bloodwork. Why no CXR initially? She had no respiratory symptoms, and her lungs were clear. Ordering a complete septic workup for every patient with a fever is neither practical nor cost effective. However, trust your instincts, thoroughly evaluate your patients, and follow up when your intuition tells you to. Even something as seemingly minor as checking that the chart has current contact information if you anticipate receiving critical test results is part of your responsibility.

- It is not reasonable, practical, or cost efficient to order extensive, expensive tests on every client.
- Trust your instincts and be thorough.

27

Referrals

This chapter describes the importance of referring clients to physicians or other specialty providers when clinical cases become complex or supersede the nurse practitioner (NP) scope of practice. Clinical examples are used for explanatory purposes, but this is not a clinical chapter. Establishing a network of qualified specialists whom you can contact any day at any time is an essential part of an NP practice. Why it is essential will be clear once you have completed this chapter.

In this chapter, you will learn:

1. The importance of referring your clients to specialty providers when indicated
2. Guidelines to determine the necessity of referring a client to a specialty provider

WHY NURSE PRACTITIONERS NEED TO REFER

Nurse practitioners should refer a client to a specialty provider any time they feel that the case may be beyond their scope of practice. What does this mean? Well, perhaps asking yourself the following question will help make this clear. If this patient was a family member, would you manage their care or would you want an expert to take over? For me, this is an extremely helpful exercise, and it may be for you, too. As a provider empowered to manage patient care, you need to find guidelines that work for you.

Nurse practitioners have a solid knowledge base and are highly qualified to manage a wide variety of medical conditions. Yet, at times, it is not realistic to manage all clients. Sometimes, a second opinion from your collaborating physician or another physician colleague is necessary. Other times, it is more appropriate for the client to seek management from an expert on a particular condition.

To support this point consider the evaluation of a client with a complicated facial laceration. I have been suturing clients for more than 15 years and even offer seminars for NP students on concepts related to suturing and suturing technique. I consider myself skillful in this procedure. However, in most cases, I elect to refer clients with facial lacerations to a plastic surgeon, because an expert with the best instruments will have the highest likelihood of successful closure to minimize scarring. Not everyone agrees with me; many NPs in primary and urgent care are comfortable performing this procedure themselves. There are some insurance plans that may, in fact, penalize primary care practices for overuse of referrals to specialty providers. The novice NP must become familiar with managed care policies and have open discussions with seasoned NPs and physicians about when referrals to other providers are indicated and, explicitly, what is in the patient's (not the insurance company's) best interest.

FAST FACTS in a NUTSHELL

Nurse practitioners should refer a client any time they feel the client's needs may be beyond the NP's level of expertise.

GUIDELINES FOR REFERRAL

An NP might refer a client to a physician specialist for a multitude of reasons that are highly dependent on the setting in which the NP is practicing, as well as his or her own level of expertise. For example, an NP working in primary care would need to use a wide variety of specialists, as he or she has general knowledge in all areas but does not specialize. Common examples of specialists to whom a primary care NP would refer clients include a dermatologist, neurologist, pulmonologist, and urologist. In contrast, an NP working in cardiology or gastroenterology might not need to refer clients to as many specialists but would refer to his or her collaborating physician when a clinical case became complex.

A friend, who is a family nurse practitioner (FNP) at a primary practice site and specializes in college health care, corrected my misconception that this population demographic was relatively healthy. I thought specialty referrals would not be a large part of the NP's responsibility. Was I wrong!

Although young adults are, for the most part, healthy, they are commonly away from home for the first time, stressed out, and not eating or sleeping properly. Some also might be engaging in high-risk activities. They present with a variety of complex health care issues, many of which are managed by NPs in the health center. Other conditions require consults with specialists, including, for example, peritonsillar abscesses (ear, nose, and throat), appendicitis (emergency/surgical consult), fractures (orthopedists), large ovarian cysts (gynecologist), corneal abrasions and foreign bodies (ophthalmologist), or thyroid masses (endocrinologist). It is also common for this population to need to consult a psychiatrist or psychologist to address mental health issues, many of which can present at this age or at the time of a new stressor. See what I mean about learning something new every day?

Physician specialists, such as neurologists, ophthalmologists, ENTs, cardiologists, pulmonologists, gastroenterologists, surgeons, dermatologists, orthopedists, gynecologists, urologists, endocrinologists, and psychiatrists, are integral partners in facilitating expert medical care for an NP's clients.

The following clinical scenario highlights the importance of referring clients to a specialty provider when appropriate. Answer the question at the end to see what you have learned.

One busy Saturday morning, a young and healthy male patient in his 20s presented with a "pimple" on his buttocks. He described it as painful, particularly with applied pressure. He denied any past medical history, trauma to the region, or history of similar lesions.

On examination, a simple infected pilonidal cyst was identified. He refused to have the cyst lanced, but agreed to a dose of an intramuscular antibiotic and to follow up in 24 hours. The case appeared rather straightforward, and my impression was that he was reliable and would return as instructed. He verbalized understanding of the importance of compliance, as well as the signs and symptoms for seeking emergent care. The case was clearly documented.

On his return the next day, he moved slowly onto the examination table, with facial grimacing on position changes. The site of infection had become much larger. There was erythema and edema, and it was extremely tender to touch. Copious amounts of foul-smelling purulent discharge poured out while the cyst was incised and drained. It was obvious that the cyst was nonresponsive to treatment and that the case was moving beyond my scope of practice.

Fortunately, I have established a network of physician specialty colleagues to whom I can refer questions and patients. Once these relationships form, you can usually reach the specialist in a reasonable amount of time. I immediately contacted a surgeon with whom I had grown comfortable and presented the case. Luckily, she was able to meet the patient directly in the emergency department.

She informed me later that day that she had brought the patient directly to the operating room, as his infection had spread so deep, so quickly, that it required immediate surgical intervention. The patient was fortunate (as was I!) that the specialist's prompt and proper evaluation and management took place in such a timely fashion. The patient followed up with me several days later. He was particularly thankful for my concern and attentiveness and for the specialist's care.

Question: What is the single most important factor in the positive outcome of this clinical case?

Answer: The NP's ability to recognize that the client's needs had gone beyond her scope of practice and her ability to identify a qualified specialist for prompt evaluation and treatment.

════════════════════════*FAST FACTS in a NUTSHELL*

Establishing a network of qualified specialists that you are able to contact at any day at any time is an essential part of effective NP practice.

28

Marketing the Role to Nurses, Employers, and the Public

This chapter presents the various ways in which nurse practitioners (NPs) can effectively market the role. NPs must demonstrate competency and confidence in promoting the role to other nurses, current and future employers, as well as the public. Barriers to marketing are described, along with ways to reduce or possibly eliminate them. Informal as well as more formal marketing strategies are discussed.

In this chapter, you will learn:

1. Why it is important for NPs to market the role
2. What barriers to marketing the role may exist, and what are strategies to minimize them
3. What are some formal, as well as informal, strategies to market the role of the NP

MARKETING THE ROLE . . . WHY, HOW, AND TO WHOM

In support of our professional role, NPs must take an active role in marketing ourselves both within and outside of the discipline of nursing. It is unfortunate that NPs still meet resistance toward the advanced practice role from other nurses. It is equally as burdensome when our physician colleagues do not support NPs practicing to the extent of our scope of practice. When physicians do not support our role, the public can become confused or question our autonomy in advanced nursing practice.

It is my belief that the best way to market our role is to practice in a thorough, holistic, comprehensive, professional, "pro-patient" manner at all times. No matter what a patient may read or hear, whether supportive of the role of the NP or not, if he or she has a positive experience that patient will come back and, perhaps more importantly, will tell a friend. NPs are the health care provider of choice in many settings and more than 900 million visits were made by NPs in the United States in 2013 (Goodread, 2014). Our patients and their families are well aware of the quality of care we provide them with. Patient recommendations are another effective way to market our role in the public eye.

FAST FACTS in a NUTSHELL

Nurse practitioners must play an active role in marketing the role to other nurses, current and future employers, and the public.

There are, of course, other more formal ways to market all that NPs offer our patients and their families. For instance, many NPs have made the decision to start their own practices. In order to be successful, these entrepreneurial colleagues must develop, perfect, and implement a business plan that includes strategies for marketing to the public all that they, as NPs, can offer. The following table provides a series of questions to get this process started:

Four P's of Marketing	Questions to Prepare Answers to:
Product	What do you do? What makes your services unique?

Four P's of Marketing	Questions to Prepare Answers to:
Place	Where can consumers find your services? What are your office hours? Are you available after hours? Do you have a website?
Price	What are your rates? Do you accept insurance? What discounts are available, if any?
Promotion	How will you advertise? Do you need to educate the public? Do you expect referrals?

Source: Rollet, J. (n. d.).

If going out on your own is part of your desired career trajectory, then I suggest you think long and hard to formulate answers to the questions posed in the preceding table. This, however, is only the first step. There are potential barriers to marketing the NP role effectively. These include, but are not limited to, ineffective strategizing, lack of clarity in differentiating what the NP can offer that others may not, inability to coordinate marketing strategy with all members of the team, and a lack of access to the consumer.

Today a savvy business owner likely will need assistance in marketing and advertising. In most instances this should include expertise in website development and maintenance as well as the proper use of social media. If the NP has not mastered these critical aspects of advertising and marketing, obtaining guidance and support from other professionals may increase the long-term success of an independent practice.

═══════════════*FAST FACTS in a NUTSHELL*

It is the responsibility of all NPs to promote the efficacy of the role and positive outcomes for our patients and their families.

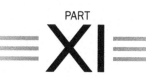

PART

XI

Economics, Policy, and Future Practice

29

Surviving Health Care Reform Today and Tomorrow

This chapter explores how nurse practitioners (NPs) can effectively contribute to the success of reform measures enacted to improve the quality and affordability of health care in the United States. Ways in which NPs can thrive throughout this evolution are presented. Issues related to how NPs are affected by this legislation are also explored.

In this chapter, you will learn:

1. How health care reform affects NP practice
2. An example of a new model to improve care
3. How NPs can adapt our role to flourish in the evolving health care system in the United States

THE DEBATE OVER HEALTH CARE REFORM

The Patient Protection and Affordable Care Act was passed in the U.S. Senate on December 24, 2009, and—after much debate—in the House of Representatives on March 21, 2010. It was signed into law by President Obama on March 23,

2010 and subsequently upheld by the U.S. Supreme Court on June 28, 2012.

Health care reform was necessary. No matter where you place yourself on the political spectrum, as a health care professional you must acknowledge that the system as it existed was a broken one. Since its rollout, the Affordable Care Act (ACA), popularly referred to as "Obamacare," has increased the numbers of insured patients and, therefore, threatens to worsen existing shortages of physicians (Greipel, 2014). This trend, coupled with the aging baby boomer population, is expected to result in a shortage of primary care physicians, in particular, which has implications for NPs (Gamble, 2014). As well as being participants in this historic transition in our nation, NPs can benefit from this evolution in modern health care through enhanced opportunities in existing settings coupled with countless possibilities and avenues to explore. The sky is the limit!

FAST FACTS in a NUTSHELL

The implementation of the ACA has increased the numbers of insured patients, worsening the current shortage of physicians and creating a wealth of new opportunities for nurse practitioners.

NEW AND EVOLVING MODELS OF CARE

The ACA is fueling reimbursement approaches that emphasize more accountable care (Japsen, 2013). One way NPs can help fulfill the growing health care needs of the population, while controlling costs and improving care, is through active participation in innovative models of care such as the patient-centered medical home (PCMH). A PCMH is a model of primary care in which a practice is redesigned to emphasize the core attributes of primary care with the goal of better coordinating care and, overall, improving patient care outcomes.

The PCMH is one example of how economic constraints and subsequent health care reform have transformed advanced nursing practice. NPs will play an integral role in the implementation of new health care models such as the PCMH. We, along with our physician colleagues and other members of the multidisciplinary team, must continue to partner in creative, innovative, and forward-thinking ways to develop new models that strive to be cost conscious, improve quality, and achieve optimal wellness for the patients we serve. Such efforts will continue to evolve as health care reform is implemented in the United States.

IMPLICATIONS FOR NURSE PRACTITIONERS

The ACA is expected to affect advanced nursing practice in a variety of ways. It is likely, however, that only a small fraction of these effects can be clearly predicted. Of course, we know that cutting costs while preserving quality is the ultimate objective. To that end, health promotion and disease prevention will be obvious key foci of health care policy, both now and as reform efforts continue to be implemented and revised. The wasteful spending of the past is no longer economically feasible. Every decision we make must ensure safety and accountability while ensuring a thoughtful, culturally competent, evidence-based, and cost-effective approach to managing patient care. This is what we, as nurses, do best.

How can the practicing NP promote positive change? Stay informed. Be active and proactive. Get involved. Be a role model. Support change. Commit to lifelong learning. Survive and thrive.

═══════════════════════════*FAST FACTS in a NUTSHELL*

The NP role will continue to thrive throughout the historic implementation of the ACA.

30

This chapter discusses the three major terminal degrees currently being offered for nurses. Some advantages of each degree are discussed. Potential flaws of each are also presented. Issues related to the importance of nurses seeking terminal degrees are described.

In this chapter, you will learn:

1. What the major differences are between the various terminal degrees in nursing are
2. Why pursuing a terminal degree in nursing is important
3. How to determine if a terminal degree is for you and, if so, which one

WHAT ARE THE VARIOUS TERMINAL DEGREES IN NURSING?

Several opportunities exist for nursing professionals to pursue a terminal degree. The terminal degrees a nurse can elect to pursue include the doctor of philosophy (PhD), doctor of education (EdD), and doctor of nursing practice (DNP). Limited doctor of nursing science (DNS; DNSc) programs are offered, however, many schools have converted these to PhD programs. Nurses must consider their own unique personal and professional goals before making the decision as to which degree best matches their anticipated career trajectory—both now and in the future.

========================= *FAST FACTS in a NUTSHELL*

The doctor of philosophy (PhD), doctor of education (EdD), and doctor of nursing practice (DNP) are the three most common terminal degrees for nursing professionals to consider.

WHY PURSUE A TERMINAL DEGREE IN NURSING?

There are numerous reasons to pursue a doctoral degree in nursing. During the historic implementation of health care reform in the United States, nurses have been called upon to assume leadership positions, advocate for our patients and their families, and promote change. In a May 2012 White House press release (Muñoz, 2012), the Obama administration stressed the central role of nurses in the health care reform effort, citing the findings of a U.S. Department of Health and Human Services report:

> *Nurses are at the center of the American health system. There are more nurses in our country than any other type of health care provider. And they do it all, from delivering preventive care to our children to helping seniors manage chronic disease. There is virtually no setting where health care is delivered where you won't find a nurse. The Affordable Care Act has given nurses a historic opportunity to improve the health of millions of Americans. The nursing profession is positioned to contribute even more than ever before to both health and health care.*

> The period of historic health care reform has given nursing professionals greater opportunities to lead, and a terminal degree promotes nurses to "sit at the table" with other members of the multidisciplinary team.

Historically, PhD- and EdD-prepared nurses have assumed academic positions in nursing education. Many conduct nursing research with the aim of disseminating evidence for practicing nurses and to contribute to the advancement of nursing education. Some of these nurses also maintain clinical practice in a variety of nursing and advanced practice nursing settings. For me, an academic track has provided the opportunity to participate in all three areas expected of me as an NP—education, research, and advanced nursing practice.

The DNP degree has been recommended as the standard for entry to advanced practice by the year 2015 by American Association of Colleges of Nursing. A nurse with a doctoral degree has parity with other disciplines such as medicine, pharmacy, physical therapy, and psychology—all which have established a practice doctorate as the standard of entry into practice. A terminal degree in nursing allows the professional nurse to develop expertise and leadership capability to, in essence, sit "at the table" in order to work effectively to enhance care and promote change along with our colleagues on the multidisciplinary team.

Specifically, a DNP degree provides nursing professionals with the unique opportunity to attain expertise through a concentration on direct care and, more specifically, research utilization for improved delivery of care, patient outcomes, and clinical systems management. The DNP degree has been developed to allow nurses to gain additional knowledge to improve practice, to strengthen leadership skills, to improve health care delivery, to enhance the status of the profession, and to achieve the overall goal of improved patient health care outcomes.

Consider the following scenario and answer the question at the end based on what you have learned in this chapter.

Carl previously practiced as a medical–surgical nurse in an acute care setting for more than 10 years. He returned for his master's degree in nursing, passed his adult–gerontology nurse practitioner (AGNP) certification exam, and accepted a position in an internal medicine practice where he has been happily employed for the past 5 years. While in graduate school, he partially funded his tuition by serving as a research assistant on a grant-funded project with a nurse faculty member and developed a passion for nursing research. For the past 2 years, he has taught several graduate-level courses in the evening for a local NP program. He is now considering doctoral studies. What terminal degree in nursing *best* matches Carl's anticipated career trajectory?

1. Doctor of philosophy (PhD)
2. Doctor of education (EdD)
3. Doctor of nursing practice (DNP)
4. Doctor of nursing science (DNS)
5. All of the above

Correct answer: 5.

Any of the terminal degrees in nursing are possible options for Carl. Carl has developed an interest in research, education, and practice. What is most important is that he pursue his nursing education to the doctoral level. Carl should begin the process of self-reflection and, perhaps, further explore his options. For example, many academic institutions do not provide tenure-track opportunities to faculty with clinical doctoral degrees so if a tenured position is his goal, Carl should research what is available in his area or consider pursuing alternate terminal degrees in nursing.

=== FAST FACTS in a NUTSHELL

Each of the terminal degrees in nursing serves a unique purpose in continuing to move the nursing profession to the forefront in today's health care system.

References

Advance Healthcare Network. (2013). 2013 National Salary Survey results. Retrieved from http://nurse-practitioners-and-physician-assistants.advanceweb.com/Features/Articles/2013-National-Salary-Survey-Results.aspx

Aktan, N. (2010). Clinical preceptoring: What's in it for me? *The Journal of the Nurse Practitioner,* 6(2), 159–160.

AMDA: The Society for Post-Acute and Long-Term Care Medicine. (n.d.). Supervision and collaboration: A review of definitions. Accessed November 20, 2014, from http://www.amda.com/advocacy/reviewdefinitions.pdf

American Association of Nurse Practitioners. (n.d.). State practice environment. Accessed November 20, 2014, from http://www.aanp.org/legislation-regulation/state-legislation-regulation/state-practice-environmen

Epocrates. Available from http://epocrates.com

Gamble, M. (2014). Whatever you want to think about nurse practitioners, there's a survey to back it up. The Daily Blog Beat. *Becker's Hospital Review.* Accessed November 20, 2014, from http://www.beckershospitalreview.com/healthcare-blog/whatever-you-want-to-think-about-nurse-practitioners-there-s-a-survey-to-back-it-up.html

Goodread. (2014). Expand the role of nurse practitioners for veterans. *Post Bulletin.*

Green, E., Wendland, J., Carver, M., Hughes, R., & Mun, S. (2012). Lessons learned from implementing the patient-centered medical home. *International Journal Telemedicine & Applications.* Epub. Doi:10.1155/2012/103685.

Greipel, N. (2014). Nurse practitioners fight for more independence. *USA Today.*

Japsen, B. (2013). Doctor shortage could ease as Obamacare boosts nurses, physician assistants. Pharma and Healthcare. *Forbes.* Accessed November 20, 2014, from http://www.forbes.com/sites/brucejapsen/2013/11/04/doctor-shortage-could-ease-as-obamacare-boosts-nurses-physician-assistants/

Muñoz, C. (May 2012). New report: Health care law invests in nurses. The White House Blog. Accessed November 20, 2014, from http://whitehouse.gov/blog/2012/05/07/new-report-health-care-law-invests-nurses

Nurse Practitioner's Prescribing Reference (NPPR). Available from http://www.haymarket.com/monthly_prescribing_reference/multi/nppr_usa_magazine/default.aspx

PDR Staff. (2014 [updated annually]). *Physician's Desk Reference.* Montvale, NJ: PDR Network.

Pocket Pharmacopeia. Available from http://www.tarascon.com/products/details.aspx/02670-2

Rollet, J. (n.d.). Business matters: Marketing your practice. Advance Healthcare Network. Accessed November 20, 2014, from http://nurse-practitioners-and-physician-assistants.advanceweb.com/Article/Marketing-Your-Practice-3.aspx

Sanford Guide to Antimicrobial Therapy. Available from http://www.sanfordguide.com/

U.S. Department of Health and Human Services, Health Resources Services Administration. (May 2012). The Obama administration's record on supporting the nursing workforce. Accessed November 20, 2014, from http://whitehouse.gov/sites/default/files/docs/nurses_report.pdf

U.S. Department of Labor, Occupational Safety and Health Administration. (n.d.). Guidelines for preventing workplace violence for health care and social service workers. Accessed November 16, 2014, from http://www.osha.gov/Publications/OSHA3148/osha3148.html

U.S. News and World Report. (2011). Nursing: Best grad schools. Accessed November 16, 2014, from http://grad-schools.usnews.rankingsandreviews.com/best-graduate-schools/top-health-schools/nursing-rankings?int=992108

U.S. News and World Report. (n.d.). Nurse practitioner: Salary. In Best Health Care Jobs. Accessed November 16, 2014, from http://money.usnews.com/careers/best-jobs/nurse-practitioner/salary

Index

additional nurse practitioner
certifications, 53
advanced practice nurses
(APNs), 5
Affordable Care Act (ACA),
172, 173
American Academy of Nurse
Practitioners (AANP),
52, 53
American Medical Association
(AMA), 145
American Nurses Credentialing
Center (ANCC), 52, 53

benefits
disability, 112
health insurance, 112
pension, 112, 113
time off, 112
"broken record technique,"
102–103
bureaucracy, 89–94
case study, 91–93
chain of command, 90
independent practice, 93–94
red tape, avoidance of, 90
role conflicts, avoidance of,
90–93

certification, 51–60
certifying organizations, 52–53
eligibility and registration
criteria for, 53–54
exams, 55–60
practice questions, 55–56
review courses, 56–58
study plan, 58–59
test readiness, 59
types of, 52–53
cheat sheets, 36–37
clinical experience, 27–29
cheat sheets, 36–37
common diagnoses and
treatments, 36–37
hours required, 34–35
immersion, 35–36
time management, 33–37
clinical preceptors, 27–31, 35
case study, 29–31
patient population, 27–28
review objectives, 29
selection of, 25–26
time with, 35
collaboration, definition, 143–144
collaborative agreement, 135–137
components of, 136–137
defining the NP role, 75